THE ART OF EXAMINING AND INTERPRET
PREPARATIONS: A LABORATORY MANUAL AND STU

Second Edition

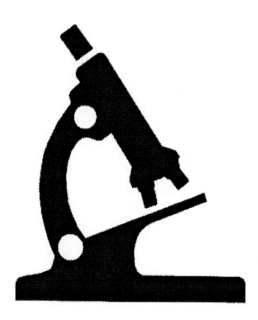

William J. Krause
Department of Pathology and Anatomical Sciences
School of Medicine
Columbia, Missouri

The Art of Examining and Interpreting Histologic Preparations:
A Laboratory Manual and Study Guide for Histology

Universal Publishers/uPUBLISH.com
Boca Raton, Florida
USA • 2004

ISBN: 1-58112-528-3

TABLE OF CONTENTS

INTRODUCTION

The examination and interpretation of tissue sections seen under the light microscope in a laboratory setting is an example of student-directed, independent problem solving. The proper reading of a histologic section is an acquired art that can only be developed through practice, close observation and repetition. This laboratory manual **was designed as a guide for students** to aid them in this endeavor. The laboratory study guide/manual was designed to be used as a supplement to any current textbook and/or atlas of Histology. **Learning objectives** provide the overall goals for each chapter. The narrative of the study guide explains how to systematically breakdown, examine and interpret each tissue and/or organ encountered, without regard to a given histologic slide from a specific slide collection. Thus, this systematic method can be used to examine and interpret histologic preparations from any collection or of any species.

The **student is encouraged to sketch, label and create a personalized atlas** while using this laboratory manual as a guide. The *vocabulary* that should be developed and used during the laboratory can be found quickly by going to the **bold face** type in the appropriate segment of the text. Each chapter contains one or more **tables** in which key structures used in the identification of a tissue/organ are presented, offering the briefest possible summary of important histologic features. As a final short review, an **appendix** provides summary tables that compare and contrasts the basic differences of several structures that are somewhat similar in general architecture.

William J. Krause
Department of Pathology and
Anatomical Sciences, School of Medicine,
University of Missouri-Columbia, Columbia, MO
August 2004

CHAPTER 1. GETTING STARTED

Have an appreciation of how a histologic preparation is made

The human body consists of two basic components: **cells** and **products of cells (extracellular materials)**. The discipline of histology is concerned primarily with the microscopic examination of these two components and how they are organized into the various tissues and organs of the body.

Obviously, if the liver, or a similar organ, were to be examined, it would be impractical to place the entire organ under a routine light microscope for study. It is not only much too large, but also opaque, therefore an examination of its microcomponents would be impossible. For this reason, and several others, a small portion of a specific tissue or organ must be **excised** from a given organ and processed for microscopic analysis. The excised tissue is placed, as soon as possible after removal, into a reagent known as a fixative. **Fixatives** act to preserve the cells and extracellular substances of tissues/organs and prevent autolytic (degenerative) changes. Although there are numerous fixatives developed for a variety of purposes, 10% buffered formalin is one of the most commonly used, routine fixatives in biology, medicine (surgical and general pathology) and biomedical research. The collected tissues, once fixed, are then **dehydrated** in graded solutions of alcohol or other dehydrating agents. Following removal of the majority of water from the collected specimens during dehydration, the tissues are cleared. **Clearing** is the process of removing the dehydrating agent and replacing it with a fluid that is miscible both with the dehydrating agent used and with the type of embedding medium chosen to make the tissue sample firm throughout. As with dehydrating agents, there are a large number of clearing reagents, the selection of which is dependent largely on the embedding medium chosen. Xylene and toluene are in common use for paraffin embedding; propylene oxide for embedding in several of the plastic embedding media. The tissue sample is next **infiltrated with** and **embedded in** the chosen embedding medium so that a firm homogeneous mass of material containing the tissue sample is obtained. Paraffin is the most commonly used embedding medium for routine preparations. The formed paraffin block, together with the contained tissue, is then sectioned (cut) into very thin slices called **sections** that normally range between 4 and 7 microns (μm) in thickness. The instrument used in cutting histologic sections is called a **microtome**. The cut sections are then transferred (mounted) onto the surface of clean glass microscope slides.

In order to prepare the **mounted sections** for staining, the paraffin embedding medium must be removed. This is accomplished by passing the slides together with their mounted sections through xylene or toluene to remove the paraffin and then through descending strengths of alcohol solutions to water, as most dyes used are in aqueous solutions. **Staining** is a process of increasing the visibility of cells by the application of dyes or by the reaction of chemical reagents with the tissue components to form visible substances. A large number of stains are available but generally only two stains are used together to provide contrasting color: one to stain the cytoplasm of cells, the other to stain the nuclei. The most common and universally used combination is the **hematoxylin and eosin (H&E) stain**. When this stain is applied to a section of tissue the **nuclei** of component cells appear **blue**; the **cytoplasm** and most **extracellular materials** a light **pink-orange**. Staining is necessary because the vast majority of cells and their extracellular materials are transparent and lack color. Only naturally occurring pigment granules such as melanin and lipofuscin would be visible on examination. The color of the dyes used during staining markedly increases the contrast of cells, their sub-components, and the associated extracellular materials. Without staining, the examination of cells and tissues with a routine light microscope would be extremely difficult. Following staining in aqueous dyes, the slides, together with their mounted, stained sections, are passed back through ascending concentrations of alcohol for dehydration, cleared with some solvent (usually xylene or toluene), and then a permanent mounting medium is put on the tissue section. A thin glass cover slip is then placed on the covering mounting medium and underlying tissue section and allowed to dry. As the histological preparation dries, the solvent evaporates from the mounting medium, which hardens, permanently cementing and sealing the tissue preparation between the glass slide and overlying cover slip. The mounting medium (balsam, damar, Permount) when dried has nearly the same refractive index as glass. After drying, the histologic section is well protected and if stored properly will usually remain unchanged for several years.

Know what you are looking for

Before examining a histologic preparation of any given tissue or organ, know something of the structure before studying it under the microscope. Such familiarity is usually acquired by carefully considering the details of the tissue/organ in question and formulating a mental image of how the structure should appear. The microscope should then be used to confirm or refute the preconceived image conceptualized. Examination of tissues and organs without prior thought and consideration of the subject usually proves frustrating and is often a waste of considerable time. Therefore, before attempting to examine any specimen for the first time with the microscope, know as much about the structure of the subject matter as possible. This information can only be acquired by attending lectures and/or reading textbooks and studying atlases.

It is **highly recommended that a small labeled sketch be made** of each section examined under the microscope using colored pencils, noting relationships and the position of specific structures and cells. This simple exercise aids in focusing concentration on the structure(s) being examined and avoids casual observation. The construction of such a labeled, personalized atlas aids in cementing the observations made in one's memory and is important in beginning to develop a mental three-dimensional image (understanding) of the tissues/organs examined from the two-dimensional image presented by the histologic preparation. The labeled sketch also serves as a highly personalized map of a specific slide for re-examination later in the exercise and is excellent for review purposes.

Making sketches

A variety of sketches should be used dependent on the structural detail needed to clearly understand a given topic. Use of several different types of sketches is suggested, the one chose dependent on the needs of the exercise.

For example: in the first exercise recommended (the identification of large cells), a simple line sketch of the entire tissue section can be used with a label showing precisely which region was used to look for and examine cells. In the case of the spinal cord, a simple outline of the tissue is all that is needed, in which nerve cells (neurons) should be identified. A supplemental sketch depicting and labeling the salient points of a neuron (cell shape, cytoplasm, position and shape of the nucleus, nucleolus and nuclear envelope) should also be used.

The other example suggested for this very important initial exercise is the identification of another of the extraordinarily large cells (ova) in the ovary. Take care to note their position in this organ and then examine the surrounding tissue for additional cells that will show a variety of different sizes and shapes. In this case, a more detailed sketch should be used to illustrate the latter points as well as focusing on the **most important aspect of the exercise:** being able to distinguish clearly between the nucleus and the cytoplasm of a given cell and to estimate nuclear and cell boundaries.

Later, sketches can be used to illustrate how cells are organized into units and how understanding such organization has led to various classification schemes, as with the classification of epithelial tissues. In this case, greater detail should be employed to illustrate cell shape, size and organization. Further details, such as modification of the cell membrane (plasmalemma) or attachment points, should also be noted.

When the histologic makeup of entire organs is considered, sketches with less cellular detail are often useful as guides as to where a particular type of tissue is located in a given organ. This is particularly true of tubular structures, the walls of which are formed by several different layers or strata. Additional accompanying detailed sketches may be needed if an important characteristic group of cells or other structures are present within the organ.

Reliable mechanics on how to examine histologic preparations (slides)

When presented with a histologic preparation (slide), the very first exercise that needs to be done is to **examine it closely with the naked eye**. A considerable amount of important information can be ascertained about the preparation using this simple exercise **before placing the slide under the microscope**. Indeed, this exercise is of such importance it should become part of the "*standard operating procedure*" for each slide examined. Initially pick up the histologic slide between the thumb and index finger and examine it by holding it up to the light or against a white background. **What to look for:** First, look at the overall nature of the preparation. Does the preparation have a doughnut configuration? If so, this immediately suggests to the viewer that the specimen being examined is tubular in nature and is being viewed in a transverse profile (hollow organs, such as blood vessels, regions of the digestive tube, tubular components of respiratory, urinary and reproductive systems, are possible organs and this list can be restricted even further if dealing only with human tissues by the size of the preparation.

Identification of the luminal surface (the lining of the internal space) as well as the external surface will be of importance when this preparation is examined further. Does the preparation have a uniform consistency and appear as a solid mass of tissue cut in the shape of a square, rectangle or wedge? If so, such a preparation usually indicates that the sample of tissue was taken from a large compact (solid) organ such as the liver, spleen, kidney or pancreas to list just a few. Once a determination has been made with regard to the shape and consistency of the tissue mounted on the slide, then examine it more carefully with regard to its staining characteristics. Of particular importance is to note if one surface (external edge or luminal surface of the doughnut-shaped configuration) stains more basophilic (light blue) than any other region in the sample of tissue being examined. Such basophilic staining usually indicates a high concentration of nuclei per unit area (nuclei stain blue with hematoxylin dye). In this way, one of the basic tissues, epithelium, can usually be located even before the histologic slide is ever viewed under the microscope. Are additional small tubular or round structures present within the tissue sample? These may indicate small blood vessels, ducts or glandular structures.

Always begin the initial examination of a histologic preparation **with the low-power (scanning) objective** and carefully **view the entire section**. This opportunity should be used to confirm or deny the observations and speculations made by direct observation with the naked eye. Add more details to the mental image being developed with regard to the preparation under examination. Note the presence or absence of more than one tissue type, patches of deeper staining, other structures present, their locations and relationships to one another and to surfaces. Only after a thorough examination with the low-power objective should the intermediate- and high-power objectives be used. Of these, the medium-power objective is the more useful for study, although more detail can be seen with the high-power objective. The disadvantage of the high-power objective is the smaller field of view and, because of this, relationships between tissues are often lost. The oil objective, if used at all, should be used only in the examination of peripheral blood and bone marrow preparations.

Since the tissues and organs of the body consist only of two elements, cells and cell products (extracellular materials) both deserve careful and thorough study. The initial exercise should be to examine the **morphology of a cell**. The following observations should be made during the examination of various cell types.

1. Shape of the cell.
2. Size of the cell (determine the position of the cell membrane).
3. Shape, size and position of the nucleus.
4. Identify the nucleolus if present in the nucleus.

It is absolutely essential that the boundary of the cell and that of the nucleus be clearly defined. Examine several cell types of various sizes and shapes to make these observations.

Large cells

Examine a section of ovary for ova. These are located in the ovarian cortex at the periphery of the ovary. The ovum represents a very large, round cell. Because of their large size, these light-staining cells can be found, by using the low-power objective, near the periphery of the ovary. After examining an ovum at low power, study it further using increased magnification. Note again the large size of the ovum, the abundant light-staining cytoplasm, and the central round nucleus separated from the cytoplasm by a well-defined nuclear membrane (envelope). Identify the **nucleolus**. It is usually round in profile and stains intensely. The nuclei of several ova may have to be examined, as these cells are so large that the plane of section may not pass through the nuclear region containing the nucleolus in all ova. Examine the remainder of the ovary and note the differences in the size and shape of the different cell types. Note that the nuclear shapes most often assume the shape of the cells being examined and that the cell membrane of most cells cannot be resolved with the light microscope. Therefore, when examining a number of tissues and organs the nuclei of component cells are often relied on in determining the orientation and shape of the cellular component and the cytoplasmic boundaries of a give cell type are estimated. The shape of the ovum is generally spherical, that of surrounding cells cube-shaped, whereas more distant cells in the ovary are spindle in shape. Examine the nuclear profile of each group of cells, noting how the shape of the nucleus reflects the shape of the cell. In addition, note the dark-staining, clumped nature of the chromatin is some nuclei. This material is referred to as **heterochromatin** and often lies adjacent to the nuclear envelope. The lighter-staining nuclear material is referred to as **euchromatin**.

The next histologic preparation that should be examined at this time is a transverse section through the spinal cord. Visual examination of the preparation will reveal an **H**-shaped area (gray matter) near the center of the preparation that surrounds a small central canal.

Examine the gray matter with the low-power objective and locate numerous, large neurons (nerve cells) found in the ventral horn. These too are exceptionally large cells with several irregularly shaped, elongated processes. Make a clear distinction between the cytoplasm, nucleus and nucleolus.

Make a small labeled sketch of several cells from these preparations illustrating the cytoplasm, the size and shape of the nucleus and the position of the nucleolus.

Cytology: structural components of a cell that can be examined with the light microscope

This laboratory guide briefly presents **a method for examining the cytologic and histologic details of human morphology** utilizing the routine H&E preparation. This preparation primarily demonstrates the nucleus and the surrounding cytoplasm of a given cell. It must be understood, however, that special staining methods can be used to demonstrate the majority of organelles, inclusions and components of the cytoskeleton within a given cell, as well as a variety of cell products and extracellular materials. These special staining methods include a variety of dyes, antibodies and other probes.

Techniques such as **immunohistochemistry**, *in situ* **hybridization** and **autoradiography** are powerful tools in demonstrating structure, secretory products, and/or messages (mRNA) **within** cells, as well as cell receptors not seen with routine preparations. The study guide focuses primarily on what can be visualized using the routine H&E preparation unless otherwise stated.

Know the basics: the basic tissues

The term **tissue** [French tissu, woven cloth] is defined as a collection of similar cells and surrounding extracellular substances that perform related functions. **Four basic tissue types** occur and these are woven together to form the fabric of all organs.

The four basic tissues are: **epithelium, connective tissue, muscle tissue** and **nervous tissue**. A thorough understanding of each of these four basic tissues is necessary before beginning an examination of individual organs or systems.

CHAPTER 2. EPITHELIUM

Epithelia consist of closely aggregated cells separated by only minimal amounts of intervening intercellular substances. Two general categories are recognized: *a lining, barrier or covering type of epithelium* organized into sheets of cells that form barriers and *glandular epithelium* modified for secretion. The sheet (barrier) form of epithelium covers the external body surface as the epidermis, lines the body cavities (pleural, pericardial, peritoneal) as well as the lumina of the cardiovascular, digestive, respiratory and urogenital systems. Thus, the majority of, if not all, substances entering or exiting the "substance of the body" must first cross an epithelial barrier. All epithelia lie on a basement membrane and are avascular. The **basement membrane** appears as a thin interphase between the epithelium and underlying connective tissue. It consists of glycoproteins, proteoglycans rich in heparin sulfate and type IV collagen. Usually the basement membrane appears only as an interphase in H&E preparations but can be demonstrated clearly using special staining techniques. As different types of epithelium are examined, a mental record should be established, keeping track of not only where a specific type of epithelium is found in a given organ but also its functional ramifications. Later, in the examination and identification of organs under the microscope, the identity and location of a specific **epithelium** is often a **key feature** in the identification.

Lining/covering (barrier) form of epithelium

Learning objectives for lining or covering epithelium:

1. Be able to locate, identify and classify the various types of epithelia in a given section of histologic material.
2. Be able to identify the various specializations of the cell membrane associated with specific epithelia.

Classification

If the covering or lining form of epithelium consists only of a single layer of cells it is termed **simple.** If two or more layers of cells are present, of which the superficial most-cells do not reach the basement membrane, the epithelium is classified as **stratified.** Once this determination has been made the next step is to determine the **geometric shape** of the **superficial-most cells** to complete the classification. Epithelial cells can be divided into three types according to their geometric shape: **squamous** (thin, flat, plate-like cells), **cuboidal** (height and width of the cell are approximately equal with the nucleus nearly touching all surfaces), and **columnar** (height of cell is greater than its width). Cells intermediate in height between cuboidal and columnar also occur and are referred to as low columnar. Thus, epithelium consisting of a single layer of cells can be classified as: simple squamous, simple cuboidal, or simple columnar. A fourth type of simple epithelium, **pseudostratified columnar**, consists of more than one cell type whose nuclei occur at different levels falsely suggesting that the epithelium is made up of two or more layers. All cells of this type of epithelium reach the basement membrane but not all reach the luminal surface.

The term **endothelium** is the specific name given to the simple squamous epithelium that lines the cardiovascular and lymph vascular systems. Examine the luminal (interior) surface of several blood vessels for this type of epithelium. The name **mesothelium** is given to the simple squamous epithelium that lines the pleural, pericardial and peritoneal cavities. Examine the external surface of a region of the stomach, jejunum or ileum for mesothelium. Examine the luminal surface of each of these organs for simple columnar epithelium. **Note:** Prior to examining these organs under the microscope, each should be examined with the naked eye. As an epithelium must lie on one surface or the other, and in the case of the gut, both, examine each of these surfaces under the microscope initially with low power for orientation prior to moving to higher power objectives for a more detailed examination.

Simple squamous epithelium

Examine the external surface of the stomach or small intestine. Note that the cells making up this form of simple squamous epithelium appear extremely attenuated, with their flattened, dense nuclei separated by considerable distances. The cytoplasm often appears only as a thin interphase between nuclei.

Simple columnar epithelium

Examine the luminal surface of the stomach for typical simple columnar epithelium. Note the basal position of the oval-shaped nuclei and that the apical cytoplasm is filled with unstained secretory granules. These can be visualized more clearly by lowering the intensity of the light and/or by dropping the condenser of the microscope. **Terminal bars** also can be seen in most preparations between the apices of adjacent cells.

They appear as minute, dense-staining short bars and represent the light microscopic appearance of the three part junctional complex (zonula occludens, zonula adherens, macula adherens) seen with the electron microscope. Examine a textbook illustration (electron micrograph) of this important junctional specialization. Examine the luminal surface of a region of small intestine. Note that it, like the stomach, is lined by a simple columnar epithelium. Carefully examine the intestinal lining epithelium and identify the **striated (microvillus) border** on the apical surface. Terminal bars also may be seen between the apices of cells forming this epithelium, as well as most other simple columnar or cuboidal epithelia.

Simple cuboidal epithelium

This type of epithelium is best seen in a section of kidney medulla, which also contains numerous tubules lined by either a simple columnar or simple squamous epithelium. Tubules lined by either simple squamous, simple columnar or simple cuboidal should be identified and compared. The nuclei of cells in a good simple cuboidal epithelium should nearly touch apical, basal and lateral cell membranes. As different tubules are examined, several examples of "low columnar" will also be encountered.

Sketch and compare tubules formed by classic examples of the three types of simple epithelia observed.

Stratified squamous epithelium

Stratified squamous is the most common of the stratified epithelia. A good example of stratified squamous is the epidermis of skin. Once again, examine the slide visually, noting the surface on which the epithelium rests, then examine it under low power. Note the presence of additional components of the skin but do not examine them at this time. Select an area of epidermis and examine it carefully under increased magnification, beginning at the basal surface. It should be quite obvious that this form of epithelium is multilayered and consists of cells that vary in their geometric shape. Cells resting on the basement membrane are columnar in shape whereas those above assume a more spindle-shaped configuration. In the outermost (superficial) layers, the cells become flat and plate-like, ie. squamous. Despite the large number of cells with different shapes, recall that the classification scheme remains based on two questions:

1. Are two or more layers of cells present, the outermost of which is not in contact with the basement membrane?

2. What is the geometric shape of the superficial-most cells?

Thus, the classification must be stratified squamous. In the case of the epidermis the superficial most cells also undergo a transformation, known as **keratinization**. As a result of this process, cells loose their nuclei and the cytoplasm becomes filled with a proteinaceous material called **keratin**. These transformed dead cells lie immediately above the intact layer of squamous cells. When this type of surface feature is present, it is usually incorporated into the terminology of the classification scheme of the epithelium. Thus, in the case of the epidermis, the complete classification of the epithelium would be **keratinized stratified squamous epithelium**. Repeat this exercise examining the epithelium lining the lumen of the esophagus. This epithelium lacks the layer of keratin on its luminal surface. Therefore, it is classified as a **non-keratinized (wet) stratified squamous epithelium**. The term wet is often used when this type of epithelium makes up a portion of a mucous membrane or lines a moist environment. Note the presence of intact nuclei in cells comprising the superficial most layer of this form of stratified squamous epithelium.

Compare the overall thickness of this epithelium with that of the epidermis and make a labeled sketch of each.

Stratified cuboidal

This type of epithelium is limited in distribution to regions of ducts from larger glands where there is a transition from a simple epithelium into a stratified epithelium. Stratified cuboidal epithelium also lines the ducts of sweat glands. Sweat glands are coiled tubes comprised of epithelial cells that extend from the base of the epidermis into the tissue of the underlying dermis and hypodermis. Because of their coiled nature, a profile of an entire sweat gland is rarely if ever encountered in sectioned material. Using the low-power objective, scan the tissue beneath the epidermis in a section of skin looking for groups of small circular and oval profiles. These cellular profiles are often encountered surprisingly deep within the underlying tissue. Two profiles will be encountered: one light staining, the other subtlety darker staining. The more darkly stained portion of the tubule is the duct region of the sweat gland. Confirm that the duct region consists of a stratified cuboidal epithelium, two cells thick, which surrounds a minute central lumen.

Sketch the duct region of a sweat gland to illustrate a stratified cuboidal epithelium.

Stratified columnar

Like stratified cuboidal, stratified columnar is restricted in its distribution confined primarily to the cavernous urethra, fornix of the conjunctiva and large excretory ducts of major glands. This epithelium is most conveniently observed in the large ducts of the parotid or submandibular gland. Examine one of these glands for the ducts only. They can be identified initially with the low-power objective by scanning the gland and looking for tubules with a very large luminal diameter. Once located, examine the wall of the duct and determine the nature of the lining epithelium. Is it stratified? Is the epithelium stratified cuboidal or stratified columnar? Both types will be encountered. Search the preparation until an example of each is found.

Make sketches of two large ducts: one lined by stratified cuboidal, the other lined by stratified columnar.

Pseudostratified columnar

This type of epithelium is a simple form of epithelium as all component cells are in contact with the underlying basement membrane, thereby satisfying the definition of a simple epithelium. The cells vary considerably in height and not all reach the luminal surface. As a result, the respective nuclei are found at different levels within this epithelium and form what appears to be two or three layers of cells, falsely suggesting stratification, hence its name. Pseudostratified columnar epithelium is somewhat restricted in its distribution, being confined primarily, but not exclusively, to the conducting portion of the respiratory system and the excurrent ducts of the male reproductive system.

Examine the trachea and epididymis for examples of this type of epithelium. Examine the luminal surface of the trachea and note the height of the epithelium and the stratified appearance due to the position of component nuclei. With the high-power objective examine the epithelium in detail beginning at the base noting the different sizes and shapes of cells forming this epithelium. Scattered within this epithelial layer are unicellular exocrine glands known as goblet cells. **Goblet cells** are sandwiched among the other epithelial cells and usually have a drinking goblet (wineglass) shape. The base of this cell is usually very narrow and contains the nucleus. The apical region is expanded due to the presence of numerous mucin granules. The latter are unstained in H&E preparations and appear as clear vacuoles. With special mucin stains they appear solid and stain brilliantly. Examine the apical surface of the pseudostratified columnar epithelium for apical specializations called cilia. **Cilia**

appear as small tufts or hair-like structures protruding from the apical cell surface. When cilia are encountered they are usually included as a prefix in the name of the epithelium. Hence, the epithelium lining the trachea would be termed a **ciliated pseudostratified columnar epithelium**.

Examination of the epididymis with the low-power objective reveals an organ that consists of several profiles of small tubules. In actual fact, the epididymis consists of one extensively coiled, elongated tubule. An appreciation of this fact at the start is of importance in developing three-dimensional mental reconstructions of images from two-dimensional images examined under the microscope. Examine the pseudostratified columnar epithelium lining the epididymal tubule at increased magnification. Note that it consists of two distinct cell types: a small basal cell and a tall columnar cell known as the principal cell. The latter have elongate, branched microvilli extending from their apical surface, which are called **stereocilia**.

Make a sketch of the ciliated pseudostratified columnar epithelium lining the trachea and compare it with an additional sketch illustrating the pseudostratified columnar epithelium lining the ductus epididymidis.

Transitional epithelium

Transitional epithelium is a stratified cuboidal type of epithelium <u>found only in the urinary system</u>. Examine this epithelium lining the interior of either the urinary bladder or ureter. Note the thickness of this epithelium and the large dome-shaped cells at the luminal surface. The latter may be binucleate.

Make a sketch of transitional epithelium from the lining of the ureter.

Specializations associated with the cell membrane of epithelial cells

Microvilli

Closely re-examine the apices of cells forming the simple columnar epithelium lining the small intestine. Note the **striated (microvillus) border** found at this location. Next, find and examine the proximal convoluted tubule of the kidney. This tubule is found only in the renal cortex (the outer region of the kidney), is the longest tubule in the cortex (therefore exhibits the most numerous tubular profiles) and is the most granular and darkly stained tubule. The apices of cells forming the proximal tubule exhibit numerous microvilli closely packed together to form the **brush border** of light microscopy.

Re-examine the **stereocilia** on the apices of the epithelial cells lining the tubule of the epididymis. Stereocilia are a thin, highly branched form of microvillus.

Cilia

Re-examine the ciliated pseudostratified columnar epithelium lining the trachea. Note that individual cilia can be seen. If the preparation is good (particularly if the embedding medium is a plastic resin of some type) numerous **basal bodies** can be visualized in the apical cytoplasm immediately beneath the cilia and appear as a dense beaded line. Examine the ciliated simple columnar epithelium lining the oviduct for the same features.

Make sketches comparing the apical specializations found on the epithelial surfaces examined above. In addition, examine several textbook illustrations of each apical specialization for their ultrastructural features.

Basal striations

Two organs that contain cells that show excellent examples of this specialization of the cell membrane are the distal convoluted tubules of the kidney cortex and the striated ducts of the submandibular gland. Re-examine the cortical region of the kidney with the low-power objective for light-staining tubules. When examined at higher magnification note that these lighter-staining epithelial cells show distinct nuclear profiles and lack the microvillus border observed in cells forming the proximal convoluted tubules.

Careful examination of the basal cytoplasm of cells forming the distal tubule will reveal faint striations. The intensity of light in the microscope may have to be decreased and/or the condenser lowered to make the basal striations more visible. With special staining techniques (iron hematoxylin - which actually demonstrates mitochondria) the basal striations are dramatic. Basal striations represent a complex infolding of the basolateral cell membrane plus a parallel arrangement of associated mitochondria. Examine a section of submandibular gland for a smaller caliber duct within the lobules of the gland. The striated ducts are intralobular ducts and appear as numerous circular profiles with wide lumina within the glandular tissue. The epithelium lining these ducts is simple cuboidal to columnar in type, is light staining and agranular. Close observation of the basal cytoplasm using the same conditions as when examining the distal convoluted tubule of the kidney will demonstrate faint basal striations within cells making up the striated ducts. **Note**: these ducts were so named because of the basal striations. Examine a textbook electron micrograph of cells from the distal convoluted tubule of the kidney for basolateral infoldings. Compare these features with those seen with the light microscope.

Make a sketch illustrating this morphological feature.

Table 1. Location of epithelia.		
Type of Epithelium	**Location**	**Specialization**
Simple squamous	Endothelium, mesothelium, thin segment of loop of Henle, rete testis, pulmonary alveoli, parietal layer of Bowman s capsule	
Simple cuboidal	Thyroid, choroid plexus, ducts of many glands, lens epithelial cells, covering surface of ovary, corneal endothelium	
Simple columnar	Surface lining epithelium of stomach, gallbladder, ducts of several glands	
	Surface lining epithelium of small and large intestines	Striated border
	Proximal convoluted tubule of kidney	Brush border
	Distal convoluted tubule of kidney	Basal striations
	Oviducts, uterus, small bronchi and bronchioles	Cilia
Pseudostratified columnar	Trachea, major bronchi, eustachian tube	Cilia
	Large excretory ducts of glands, portions of male urethra	
	Epididymis	Stereocilia
Stratified squamous	Esophagus, epiglottis, corneal epithelium, vagina	
	Epidermis of skin	Keratin
Stratified cuboidal	Ducts of sweat glands, large ducts of salivary glands	
Stratified columnar	Large ducts of glands, cavernous urethra	
Transitional	Restricted to urinary system: renal calyces to urethra	

Glandular forms of epithelium

Glands are comprised of epithelial cells specialized to synthesize and secrete a product of some type. A variety of different criteria can be used in the classification of glands. The simplest classification scheme is to divide the glands into **endocrine** (secretion into the lymph/vascular system) and **exocrine** (secretion onto an epithelial surface or into a duct) glands. A consideration of the endocrine glands will be presented later as a specific topic.

Exocrine glands can be classified further as to whether they are unicellular or multicellular. A classic example of a **unicellular exocrine gland** is the goblet cell. Re-examine the epithelium lining the intestine and trachea for goblet cells. Carefully study this cell, paying particular attention to its overall shape, position of the nucleus, and the apical accumulation of secretory (mucin) granules. Recall that the mucin granules, although unstained with the H&E preparation, can usually be visualized by lowering the intensity of the light and by lowering the condenser.

The majority of glands are **multicellular exocrine glands**. Multicellular glands can assume a wide variety of morphologies. They may occur as a small group of secretory cells that lie wholly within an epithelial layer, clustered about a small lumen. These are called **intraepithelial glands**. An example of this glandular organization can be found in the non-keratinized stratified squamous epithelium lining the penile urethrae of the male reproductive system. Examine this lining epithelium. The intraepithelial glands (glands of Littr) appear as clusters of clear or light-staining cells within the more darkly stained lining epithelium. The nuclei of component secretory cells are generally compressed to the base and the apical portion of the cell is filled with unstained mucin secretory granules. A somewhat similar glandular organization is the **secretory sheet**. In this case, the cells form a continuous epithelial layer. An example of this type of multicellular gland is the gastric lining epithelium of the stomach. This glandular form consists of a simple columnar, mucous secreting epithelium that secretes directly into the lumen of the stomach. Examine this epithelial form again.

The majority of multicellular, exocrine glands secrete into a ductal system. These are classified according to the morphology of the ducts and how their secretory cells are arranged to form the secretory portion of the gland. If the **duct branches** the gland is classified as **compound**; if the **duct does not branch** the gland is classified as **simple**. The secretory cells of the gland may be arranged into **tubules** and/or **acini** (**alveoli**) (berry-like end pieces). Subsequent classification depends on the shape and configuration of the secretory unit and whether these portions also branch. Thus, **simple glands** can be classed as simple tubular, simple coiled tubular, simple branched tubular, or simple branched acinar (alveolar). **Compound glands** are subdivided into compound tubular, compound acinar and compound tubuloacinar (compound tubuloalveolar).

Learning objectives for glandular epithelia and exocrine glands:

1. Be able to classify glands according to their histologic organization, type of material secreted and manner in which material is secreted.

Simple glands

Simple tubular glands

Examine a section of colon with the low-power objective. Find and examine the luminal surface of this organ and note that it is lined by a simple columnar epithelium. Observe the large number of goblet cells. Identify tubular invaginations that extend from this epithelium into the underlying tissue. These are the simple tubular glands (intestinal glands) of the colon. The epithelium forming the walls of these glands is the same as that lining the surface. If the plane of section through the wall of the colon is at an oblique angle, the glands may appear as isolated oval or circular collections of columnar cells surrounding a tiny lumen. If the glands are cut parallel to their long axis, the lumen of the gland can be traced to that of the colon. Next, examine a section of small intestine. In the small intestine, the simple tubular intestinal glands open between the bases of fingerlike extensions of tissue covered by simple columnar (intestinal) epithelium called villi. Compare the glands at this location with those of colon. Note the numerous mitotic figures within the epithelium forming these glands.

Draw and label a sketch of these structures, including the location of the simple tubular intestinal glands in a section of colon and small intestine.

Simple coiled tubular glands

Re-examine the section of skin for eccrine sweat glands as an example of a simple coiled tubular gland. Using the low power objective examine the deep subcutaneous tissue far beneath the overlying keratinized stratified squamous epithelium for these glands. The duct is long, extending from the surface epithelium to deep within the underlying tissue.

The secretory portion ends as a highly coiled structure similar to that of a coiled snail shell. A section through such a unit results in several circular cross-sectional profiles. These are lined by lightly stained simple columnar epithelial cells. The ducts are more darkly stained and lined by stratified cuboidal epithelium.

Simple branched alveolar glands

Continue to examine the preparation of skin for sebaceous glands. These glands are classified as simple branched alveolar glands and are almost always associated with hair follicles. The latter are invaginations of the epithelium into underlying tissue that produce and contain hair shafts. Study the sebaceous glands carefully. Note the presence of large flask-shaped secretory units, the alveoli. Alveoli of sebaceous glands consist of large cells filled with small lipid droplets, which gives them a light-staining, vacuolated appearance. Note that two or three alveoli drain into a single, short unbranched duct lined by stratified squamous epithelium. The duct empties into the lumen of an adjacent hair follicle. The overall three-dimensional shape of these glands is similar to a three or four leaf clover.

Sketch, label and compare a simple coiled tubular sweat gland with a simple branched alveolar (sebaceous) gland of the skin (integument).

Simple branched tubular glands

Study a section taken from the pyloric region of the stomach. Identify the gastric pits. These are tubular invaginations of the gastric surface lined by simple columnar epithelium that extend into the underlying tissue. Emptying into the bottoms of the gastric pits are the pyloric glands, an example of simple branched tubular glands. Cells forming these glands have basal nuclei and a light/clear supranuclear cytoplasm that contains mucin granules. Note that in this glandular form, the duct remains unbranched (simple) and that it is the secretory tubule that branches.

Sketch and label the subcomponents of a simple branched tubular gland from the pyloric region of the stomach.

Compound glands

Compound tubular glands

Examine a slide of the duodenum and scan it carefully. Find the location of numerous light-staining, secretory tubules of the duodenal (Brunner s) glands within the intestinal wall. These glands are found in the tissue beneath the bottoms of the simple tubular intestinal glands examined earlier in other regions of the intestinal tract. Now examine the duodenal glands at increased magnification. The terminal portions (secretory units) of the duodenal glands are branched, coiled and of uniform diameter. Component cells are light staining with basally positioned nuclei. The branching ducts are lined by a similar appearing epithelium to that forming the secretory units. The ducts of the duodenal glands unite with the bottoms of the overlying intestinal glands. Note the differences in the lining epithelium between glands where this transition occurs.

Sketch and label a duodenal gland including its association with an overlying simple tubular intestinal gland.

Compound tubuloacinar (alveolar) glands

This type of gland represents the most common glandular organization of the compound glands. As an example, study a section of the submandibular (submaxillary) gland with the low-power objective identifying several important features. The gland is organized into lobes and lobules. These glandular subdivisions are limited by fibers of the surrounding connective tissue. Next identify the duct system. The ducts can be recognized by their round profiles, wide lumina, and the light-staining cytoplasm of component cells. The epithelial lining is usually simple cuboidal or simple columnar although stratified forms of both types can be found on occasion lining the very large ducts. Note that two categories of ducts can be recognized: intralobular ducts and interlobular ducts. The former occurs **within** the lobules and in the submandibular gland are the most numerous. The interlobular ducts are larger and occur **between** lobules. The lining epithelium is usually simple cuboidal or simple columnar. Can basal striations be observed with increased magnification? Because the branched ductal system of the submandibular is well developed, numerous profiles of the ductal system are observed. Carefully examine the apices of cells forming the ductal epithelium. Note the minute, dense staining points between cell apices. These are terminal bars. Next, examine the secretory units of the submandibular gland and observe that two markedly different cell types makeup the tubules and acini (alveoli) of this gland. The most numerous are **serous cells**. Serous cells are characterized by a dark staining cytoplasm filled with numerous, distinct secretory granules. The basally positioned nuclei usually exhibit a round or oval profile. The less numerous cell type making up scattered tubules is the **mucous cell**. These cells are characterized by a white (clear) cytoplasm of frothy appearance. The latter is filled with unstained mucin granules.

Nuclei appear as darkly stained, compressed profiles positioned adjacent to the basal cell membrane. Some serous cells are organized into small units called **demilunes** that cap terminal regions of the scattered mucous tubules.

When both serous and mucous cell types make up the secretory units of a gland, the gland is often referred to as a **mixed gland**.

Sketch and label the subcomponents of a lobe from the submandibular gland.

It is important to realize from the onset that the connective tissues are classified according to the *type* and ***arrangement*** of the ***extracellular materials*** rather than features of the cellular components, as is true of epithelium. General connective tissues are classified as loose or dense according to whether the extracellular materials are loosely or tightly packed. **Loose** connective tissue can be subdivided further on the basis of special constituents such as adipose (fatty) tissue or a concentration of specific extracellular fibers. **Dense** connective tissue can be subdivided according to whether the extracellular fibers are randomly distributed (dense irregular connective tissue) or orderly arranged (dense regular connective tissue).

Loose (areolar) connective tissue

Areolar connective tissue is a loosely arranged connective tissue that is widely distributed throughout the body. It consists of three extracellular fibers (collagen, reticular, elastic) in a thin, almost fluid-like, ground substance. The latter is not preserved in routine preparations and accounts for some, but not all, of the spacing observed between the fibrous and cellular components. Areolar connective tissue forms the **stroma** that binds organs and the components of organs together. It forms helices about the long axes of expandable tubular structures, such as the gastrointestinal tract and other visceral organs, the ducts of glands, and blood vessels.

Fibers of connective tissue

Learning objectives for connective tissue fibers:

1. Be able to identify and distinguish between the three types of connective tissue fibers.
2. Be able to classify general connective tissues according to the arrangement of their extracellular fibers.

Collagen fibers are present in all connective tissues, vary in thickness from 1 to 10 μm and are of undefined length. In H&E preparations they stain a pink or pink-orange color. Because of the proteinaceous subcomponents these fibers, dependent on the dye used in staining, they can also be stained blue, green, yellow or red. Examine the dermis of skin (that region underlying the keratinized stratified squamous epithelium [epidermis]) for collagen fibers. Note the variation in size and the wavy, homogeneous appearance of the pink-orange staining collagen fibers. The majority of oval, densely staining nuclei in the field are those of associated **fibroblasts** that secrete and maintain the collagen fibers. The extent of the fibroblast cytoplasm usually cannot be seen in H&E preparations and what is actually visualized are fibroblast nuclei. Examine the external surface of a medium-sized (named) vessel for collagen fibers and fibroblasts. If available, examine a spread preparation of loose areolar connective tissue for collagen fibers and fibroblasts. The advantage of this type of preparation (usually a portion of a mesentery) is that it is not a section of tissue but rather an intact tissue, which is thin enough to allow the transmission of light. Examine the fibroblasts carefully, first noting their oval-shaped nuclei and then their associated cytoplasm. In these preparations the extent of the fibroblast cytoplasm can often be traced for considerable distances. Note that the fibroblasts lie immediately adjacent to, or on, collagen fibers, which stain lightly (a light pink in most preparations). Close observation of some fibroblast nuclei will reveal a light appearing strip crossing the blue-stained fibroblast nuclei. These strips are collagen fibers as seen against the stained chromatin background of the fibroblast nuclei. Return to a section of skin and re-examine the dermis with low power. Note, once again, that it forms a thick interwoven layer beneath the overlying epithelium. At increased levels of magnification note that the abundant thick, collagenous fibers are <u>interwoven</u> to form a compact network. The dermis is a classic example of **dense irregular connective tissue**. Next, a longitudinal section of tendon or ligament should be examined in detail. Note the regular, precise arrangement of collagen fibers into bundles that run parallel to one another. Fibroblasts are the primary cell type present and occur in rows parallel to the bundles of collagen fibers. Fibroblast nuclei usually are the only feature of these cells visualized and appear elongate and densely basophilic. Tendons and ligaments are classic examples of **dense regular connective tissue**.

Sketch and label the subcomponents of a region of dermis and tendon (or ligament). Illustrate the arrangement of collagen fibers and their association with fibroblasts. Examine an electron micrograph from a textbook illustrating the fact that each collagen fiber (type I) consists of banded unit fibrils, the smallest morphologically defined unit of collagen.

Elastic fibers appear as thin, homogeneous strands that are smaller and of more uniform size than collagen fibers. Usually elastic fibers cannot be distinguished easily in routine H&E preparations and require special stains (orcein or Verhoeff's elastic stain) to make them visible.

If a spread preparation of loose areolar connective tissue stained to demonstrate elastic fibers is available, examine it carefully and note darkly stained, variously sized, thin cylindrical fibers coursing across the field. These are elastic fibers. Look for an elastic fiber that has been broken. Because of their elastic properties, broken fibers will form a highly undulated snarl much like broken elastic fibers of clothing (eg. stockings). If a specifically stained preparation is not available, elastic fibers can be visualized to some degree using the same morphological criteria as demonstrated by special staining. However, in this case the elastic fibers stain the same color as collagen fibers but are narrower (thread-like), smooth and homogeneous in appearance, and of more uniform diameter than collagen fibers.

Examine a section of a named (muscular) artery for elastic tissue. Locate the lumen of the vessel and examine the region immediately beneath the lining endothelium. Note the highly scalloped, homogeneous layer of elastic tissue (the internal elastic lamina) at this location. If the vessel is specifically stained for elastin, move through the vessel wall and examine it for other dark-staining elastic fibers of various sizes. Return to the vessel interior. The internal elastic lamina is not a fiber *per se* but a thick homogeneous sheet of elastin. Now, and in the future, when additional arteries are encountered in routine H&E preparations, examine these vessels for the **internal elastic lamina**. In routine preparations this highly scalloped appearing membrane, although stained similar to collagen, has a slightly different refractive index. The appearance of the elastin can be made more visible by dropping the condenser of the microscope. Use the known position to locate and examine the negative image of the internal elastic lamina using this technique. Examine sections of any other tissue specially stained to demonstrate elastic fibers. Examine them in both longitudinal and transverse profiles. Note again the smooth, homogeneous nature of these darkly stained fibers. They often give a "copper wire-like" appearance when seen in sections of tissue.

Reticular fibers, like elastic fibers, are not seen in routinely prepared sections but can be demonstrated with silver stains or by the periodic acid-Schiff's (PAS) procedure. These are small fibers that form delicate networks and are a major component of the **stroma** that binds the cells of tissues and organs together. The most commonly used organs to demonstrate reticular fibers are the liver, kidney, spleen and lymph node where these fibers are especially prominent. With silver-stained preparations the reticular fibers stain black. Note the fine delicate network of fibers supporting the cellular components (**parenchyma**) of these organs.

Make a sketch of reticular fibers and their association with parenchymal elements. Compare these fibers with a sketch of elastic fibers.

Table 2. Key histologic features of connective tissue fibers.

Fiber type	Light microscopic appearance	Primary locations
Collagen fibers (type I collagen)	Coarse fibers 0.5-10.0μm in diameter, indefinite length, stain with protein dyes	Tendon, ligament, dermis, fascia, capsules, sclera, bone, dentin
Reticular fibers (type III collagen)	Delicate network of fine fibers, must be stained specifically to be demonstrated, usually by a reduction of silver or the periodic acid Schiff s (PAS) staining reaction	Stroma of lymphatic organs, bone marrow, glands, and adipose tissue
Elastic fibers	Smooth, homogeneous fibers of varying diameter, must be stained specifically to demonstrate well (orcein or Verhoeff s stain)	Dermis, lung, arteries, organs that expand

Cells of connective tissue

General connective tissue may contain a wide variety of cell types. Some are indigenous (residents) of connective tissues; others are transients and migrate to and from the general connective tissue from the vasculature.

Learning objectives for connective tissue cells:

1. Be able to distinguish and identify the following cell types (both indigenous and transient cells) found within connective tissues: fibroblasts, macrophages, plasma cells, fat cells, mast cells, neutrophils, eosinophils and lymphocytes.

Indigenous cells

Fibroblasts are the most common of the connective tissue cell types. They are large, spindle-shaped cells with elliptical nuclei. The boundaries of the cell are not seen in most routine preparations and the morphology and staining intensity of the nuclei vary with the state of activity. Active fibroblasts exhibit plump, light-staining nuclei; nuclei of inactive fibroblasts appear narrow and densely stained. Re-examine preparations of dermis, tendon (ligament) and areolar connective tissue and compare fibroblast nuclei.

 Macrophages are abundant in general areolar connective tissue. They are commonly described as irregularly shaped cells with blunt cytoplasmic processes and ovoid or indented nuclei that are smaller and stain more deeply than those of fibroblasts. In actual fact, unless macrophages show evidence of phagocytosis, they are difficult to distinguish from fibroblasts. If special preparations are available, utilizing tissues from animals injected with India ink or trypan blue, examine the areolar connective tissue or liver preparations for cells that have phagocytized the materials injected. These will be macrophages. One location in which to examine macrophages in a "natural" setting is the center (medulla) of lymph nodes. Examine a routinely prepared lymph node under low power. Note that its central region is lighter staining and consists of anastomosing cords of cells separated by wide spaces. Examine the cords of cells and the adjacent spaces carefully for large rounded cells with brown-gold colored particulate material within their cytoplasm. These are macrophages.

 Continue to look carefully within the interior of the medullary cords of the lymph node and note numerous **plasma cells**. These cells appear somewhat "pear-shaped" with small eccentrically placed nuclei in which the heterochromatin is arranged into coarse blocks forming a **clock face pattern**. The cytoplasm is basophilic and a weakly stained or light area of cytoplasm often appears adjacent to the nucleus on the side facing the greatest amount of cytoplasm. This light-staining area is referred to as a **negative Golgi image**. If available, examine a section of lactating breast. The connective tissue surrounding the secretory units of this gland often contains numerous plasma cells. Plasma cells also are present in large numbers in the connective tissue (lamina propria) of the intestinal tract. Examine the connective tissue that lies between adjacent intestinal glands for both plasma cells and small lymphocytes. The latter show a round, dense nucleus and only a scant rim of cytoplasm.

 Fat cells are specialized for synthesis and storage of lipid. Individual fat cells may be encountered throughout the loose areolar connective tissue or may accumulate in large numbers to form fat (adipose) tissue. In routine sections, fat cells appear large, round and empty due to the loss of a stored central lipid droplet during tissue preparation. The remaining cytoplasm appears only as a thin rim around a large empty central space and if the nucleus is encountered in these large cells, it lies flattened on one side of the cell. Groups of fat cells have the appearance of chicken wire or a honeycomb. Fat cells are abundant in the hypodermis of skin - that region of tissue lying beneath the dermis. Fat cells are also common in the loose areolar connective tissue around the perimeter of a lymph node. If the lymph node preparation has been stained to demonstrate reticular fibers, examine the delicate network of reticular fibers enveloping each fat cell.

 Mast cells are large, ovoid cells 20 - 30 μm in diameter with large granules that fill the cytoplasm. The nucleus is oval or round in shape and centrally located. Mast cells are present in variable numbers in loose connective tissue and often accumulate along small blood vessels. Examine a mesentery or areolar spread preparation for these large granulated cells. The granules can be stained different colors depending on the dye used. In tissues embedded in a plastic resin and stained with H&E, mast cell granules stain a light red color. If sections of this type are available, examine sections of the stomach and intestinal tract. In either organ the outer supporting muscular wall and adjacent connective tissue components should be examined for mast cells. They will appear as oval-shaped cells or cytoplasmic fragments of cells packed with coarse red-orange granules.

Transient cells derived from blood

Variable numbers of **leukocytes** constantly migrate into the connective tissues from the blood to carry out their specialized functions. **Neutrophils** are one type of leukocyte characterized by a multilobed nucleus and a faintly pink-staining cytoplasm. They are generally round in shape. Most often, the multilobed nucleus is the only prominent feature recognized when these cells are encountered in a section of general connective tissue. **Eosinophil** leukocytes also exhibit multilobed nuclei and are characterized by bright red (eosinophilic)-staining granules within the cytoplasm. **Lymphocytes** are smaller leukocytes (5 - 7 μm in diameter) characterized by a central, round nucleus surrounded by a thin rim of cytoplasm. In tissue, groups of lymphocytes appear only as collections of round, dark staining nuclei. Examine the outer, more darkly stained region (cortex), of a lymph node and thymus for these small darkly stained leukocytes. Examine the lighter-staining central region (medulla) of the thymus for mast cells and eosinophils.

Sketch and compare the various cell types encountered in general connective tissue.

As plasma cells and lymphocytes are closely related, how do they differ morphologically?

Questions:

In sections of plastic embedded material stained with H&E, the cytoplasmic granules of both mast cells and eosinophil leukocytes stain red. How can these two cell types be distinguished from one another? Clue: consider their size and the nuclear profiles.

Table 3. Key cytologic features of cells found in general areolar connective tissue.		
Cell types	**Nuclear characteristics**	**Cytoplasmic characteristics**
Indigenous cells		
Fibroblasts	Oval, centrally placed, staining intensity variable depending on activity	Elongate, spindle- or stellate-shaped cell; usually not clearly distinguished is sectioned material
Unilocular fat cells (white fat)	Usually compressed at edge of cell, staining variable	Forms a thin rim around a single, large central lipid droplet
Multilocular fat cells	Central, spheroid, light staining	Numerous lipid droplets, abundant mitochondria
Mast cells	Central, spheroid to ovoid, may show abundant heterochromatin	Filled with secretory granules
Macrophages	Large, ovoid, most frequently indented	Light staining, contains phagocytosed material
Plasma cells	Usually eccentric, spheroid; heterochromatin clumps may form clock face	Basophilic, slate gray in color; may show negative Golgi image
Transient cells		
Neutrophils	Polymorphonuclear, 3-5 lobes common, chromatin dense	Light lilac staining granules
Eosinophils	Polymorphonuclear, 2-4 lobes common, chromatin dense	Bright red-orange granules fill the cytoplasm
Lymphocytes	Single, spheroid, abundant heterochromatin	Thin rim, light transparent blue staining

Cartilage

The classification of cartilage into hyaline, elastic or fibrous is based on the differences in the abundance and type of fiber within the matrix. **Fibers** and the **ground substance** constitute the **matrix** of cartilage.

Learning objectives for cartilage:

1. Be able to identify the three types of cartilage (hyaline, elastic and fibrous (fibro) cartilage) and their subcomponents.

Hyaline cartilage is the most common type of cartilage and forms the cartilages of the nose, larynx, trachea, bronchi, costal cartilages and the articular cartilages of joints. Examine the trachea or another tissue that contains hyaline cartilage. In the trachea, hyaline cartilage appears as a large homogeneous mass of tissue with a glassy appearance. The matrix appears homogeneous because the ground substance and the collagen fibers (type II) embedded within it have the same refractive index. Scattered within the light-staining, homogeneous cartilage matrix are small spaces called **lacunae**. These spaces contain the cells of cartilage known as **chondrocytes**. Chondrocytes generally conform to the shape of the lacunae in which they are housed. Note that deep within the interior of cartilage the cells and their lacunae usually exhibit a rounded profile whereas near the surface (edge) they are elliptical and flattened with the long axis oriented parallel to the surface. Near the center, chondrocytes often occur in small clusters called **isogenous groups**. The more intensely stained matrix immediately around chondrocytes is termed the **territorial matrix**. The less densely stained intervening matrix is called the **interterritorial matrix**. Except for the free surfaces of articular cartilages, hyaline cartilage is enclosed in a specialized connective tissue membrane (sheath) called the **perichondrium**. The outer region of the perichondrium is formed by a well-vascularized, dense irregular connective tissue. The region adjacent to the cartilage matrix is more cellular and the transition into cartilage is imperceptible. The perichondrial cells adjacent to the cartilage retain the capacity to form new cartilage.

Elastic cartilage is more flexible than hyaline cartilage and is found in the epiglottis, external ear, auditory tube and some of the small laryngeal cartilages. Elastic cartilage differs from hyaline cartilage chiefly in that the matrix contains an abundance of elastic fibers. Elastic fibers form a dense, closely packed mesh that obscures the ground substance deep within the cartilage, but, beneath the perichondrium, the fibers form a loose network and are continuous with those of the perichondrium. The elastic fibers of elastic cartilage, like those elsewhere, need to be specifically stained to be well demonstrated. Identify the perichondrium, matrix, lacunae and chondrocytes in elastic cartilage and compare them with similar structures found in hyaline cartilage.

Fibrous (fibro-) cartilage occurs in the symphysis pubis, intervertebral discs, in some articular cartilages and at sites of attachment of major tendons to bone. Fibrous cartilage **lacks a perichondrium** and merges into bone, hyaline cartilage or dense fibrous connective tissue. Fibrous cartilage represents a transition between cartilage and dense connective tissue. Typical chondrocytes enclosed in lacunae are found but only a small amount of ground substance is present in the immediate vicinity of the cartilage cells. **Chondrocytes** may **occur singly, in pairs or in short rows between** well defined bundles of **dense collagen fibers (type I)**.

Make a sketch of the three types of cartilage and label their subcomponents.

Bone

Two forms of bone can be recognized by visual inspection: compact (dense) bone and cancellous (spongy) bone.

Compact (dense) bone forms the solid, continuous mass that forms the perimeter of the named bones of the skeleton. **Cancellous (spongy bone)** is formed by an interlacing network of bony rods called **trabeculae**. These branch and unite to form a three-dimensional system of bony rods separated by small communicating spaces that form the marrow cavity. Bone is covered, except over articular surfaces and where tendons and ligaments attach, by a fibroelastic connective tissue membrane called the **periosteum**. A similar, less fibrous membrane, the **endosteum**, lines the marrow cavity.

Learning objectives for bone:

1. Be able to identify bone tissue and its subcomponents.

Compact bone

The initial examination of compact bone should be done using a ground preparation rather than a histological section of bone as the microscopic detail of the **matrix** is much more pronounced.

Bone is characterized by the arrangement of its matrix into layers called **lamellae**. Small, ovoid spaces, the **lacunae**, occur rather uniformly between and within lamellae, each housing a single bone cell called an **osteocyte**. Minute tubules called **canaliculi** radiate from each lacuna, penetrate and cross lamellae to join with canaliculi from adjacent lacunae. In compact bone, lamellae show three configurations. In transverse sections, most are arranged concentrically into several cylindrical units, much like growth rings of a tree. The concentrically arranged lamellae surround a central space known as a **Haversian canal**. Each unit, consisting of 8 to 15 concentric lamellae that surround the central Haversian canal, is referred to as an **Haversian system** or **osteon**. Portions of additional lamellae can also be visualized filling in the regions between osteon units. These are called **interstitial lamellae**. At the external surface, several lamellae course around the entire external circumference of the bone. These are called the **outer circumferential lamellae**. A similar but less well developed system of lamellae (one or two lamellae in thickness) lines the interior surface adjacent to the marrow cavity and these are referred to as the **inner circumferential lamellae**. Close inspection of individual osteons will reveal that they are outlined by a refractile line of modified matrix, the **cement line**. Note that the cement lines are not traversed by canaliculi. It must be emphasized that when viewing a preparation of ground bone (pieces of bone ground thin enough to permit the transmission of light) **only the matrix is observed** and the lacunar spaces and canaliculi within it. To visualize the cells of bone and the vascularized connective tissues associated with bone (periosteum and endosteum) a decalcified, histologically cut and stained section of bone must be used. Identify all the features observed previously using the preparation of ground bone in a histologic section of bone. Note that the matrix, at initial inspection, appears smooth, homogeneous and stains a light pink-red. It appears similar to hyaline cartilage. On closer observation, however, note the organization of the matrix. **Lacunae** contain **osteocytes** and are organized in a circular pattern around a **central Haversian canal**. Using low power, scan the section and identify several osteon units. By lowering the intensity of light and lowering the condenser note that the lamellae are crossed by fine, unstained canaliculi which can be traced to lacunae and give the latter a very irregular shape. Carefully examine these features under high power. Use of the fine focus adjustment, focusing back and forth through the section, may be required to see these structures. Carefully examine several Haversian canals. Note that they contain a delicate connective tissue that contains at least two small blood vessels. In well-preserved specimens a layer of

flattened cells lines the limiting wall of the Haversian canal. These cells have osteogenic potential, ie, they can transform into bone-forming cells, osteoblasts, and can produce bone during the remodeling process. In addition, note the differences in diameter of the Haversian canals. Why is this? Is it related to the remodeling process? The delicate vascular connective tissue found within the Haversian canals is an extension of the endosteum, which also lines the marrow cavity. Compare the **endosteum** with the much thicker **periosteum** covering the external surface of bone. The outermost layer of the periosteum is dense irregular connective tissue with abundant collagen fibers, some elastic fibers, scattered fibroblasts and a network of blood vessels. The region of periosteum closest to bone is more cellular and consists of a loosely arranged connective tissue. Fibroblast-like cells immediately adjacent to the bone matrix are often called bone-lining cells or **osteoprogenitor cells**. If stimulated, they assume a cuboidal shape and synthesize and lay down new bone matrix. If this occurs these cells are termed **osteoblasts**. Some blood vessels leave the periosteum and enter the bone through **Volkmann s canals**. These are transverse canals that penetrate the bone from the endosteal and periosteal surfaces. Haversian canals on the other hand follow a longitudinal course parallel to the long axis of the bone and lie within osteons. Note that Volkmann s canals are not surrounded by concentric lamellae. Blood vessels passing through Volkmann s canals unite with those within the Haversian canals and link vessels in the marrow cavity and periosteum to the Haversian system. Large bundles of collagen fibers (**Sharpey s fibers**) enter the outer circumferential lamellae from the periosteum and firmly anchor the periosteum to bone. Re-examine both preparations of bone for both Volkmann s canals and Sharpey s fibers.

Sketch and label both a ground bone preparation and a section of decalcified bone. Compare and contrast the advantages and disadvantages of each preparation.

In addition to osteocytes, two other cell types are directly related to bone: osteoblasts and osteoclasts. Both are most easily found in young or developing bone and should be examined in detail.

Developing bone can form directly in a primitive connective tissue (mesenchyme) by a process known as intramembranous ossification or by replacement of a pre-formed hyaline cartilage model, the process of which is called endochondral ossification.

Learning objectives for developing bone:

1. Be able to describe the process associated with membrane bone formation and be able to identify the microscopic detail associated with a developing membrane bone.
2. Be able to describe the process associated with endochondral bone formation and be able to identify the microscopic detail associated with a developing endochondral bone.

Intramembranous ossification

Flat bones of the cranium and part of the mandible develop by intramembranous ossification and, as a result, are often referred to as **membrane bones**. Examine a section of forming membrane bone at low power and note that much of the bone is of the cancellous, or spongy, type. Carefully examine several trabeculae of the cancellous bone at higher power. Note the layer of low cuboidal, basophilic cells covering the external surface of each trabecula. These are **osteoblasts**. Examination of the interior of a trabecula will reveal **lacunae with osteocytes**. In the same region note a thin layer of bone matrix immediately adjacent to the cuboidally shaped osteoblasts that stains lighter than the remainder of the trabecular bone matrix. This layer of unmineralized matrix is called **osteoid**. After a short period it becomes mineralized to form true bone. As new osteoblasts are recruited from osteoprogenitor cells, which resemble fibroblasts, in adjacent mesenchymal tissue, they produce osteoid and eventually become enveloped in their own matrix. When this occurs the osteoblasts are termed osteocytes. With development, the trabeculae continue to thicken by the addition of new bone on their external surface (appositional growth) and the spaces between some trabeculae are gradually obliterated. As bone growth encroaches on vascular spaces within the surrounding mesenchymal connective tissue, matrix is laid down in irregular, concentric layers around blood vessels to form **primary osteons**. The entrapped blood vessels and connective tissue form the contents of the developing, primitive Haversian canals. These newly formed osteon units then undergo remodeling.

Identify and sketch several fields comparing one with the other and envision primary osteon formation.

Endochondral bone formation

Bones of the extremities, pelvis, face, base of skull and vertebral column result from endochondral bone formation, a process that involves simultaneous removal of a precursor hyaline cartilage model and formation of bone matrix. Cartilage does not contribute directly to the formation of bone but much of the process is concerned with the removal of the cartilage precursor. Initial indications of ossification of a long bone occur at the center of the cartilage model in the shaft or diaphysis. In this area, the primary ossification center, chondrocytes hypertrophy, their lacunae expand and the matrix between adjacent lacunae is reduced to thin, fenestrated partitions. Simultaneously, the perichondrium becomes more vascular and assumes an osteogenic function. A thin layer of bone called the **periosteal collar** forms around the perimeter of the altered cartilage and acts as a temporary splint. Blood vessels from the former vascularized perichondrium (now best termed periosteum) invade the degenerating cartilage as a **periosteal bud**. The connective tissue sheath that accompanies the invading blood vessels contains cells with osteogenic properties. As the cartilage matrix breaks down, lacunar spaces are opened up, become confluent, and narrow tunnels in the calcified cartilage matrix are formed. Blood vessels grow into these tunnels bringing with them osteogenic cells that align themselves on the surfaces of the calcified cartilage. The latter differentiate into osteoblasts and begin to lay down new bone matrix (osteoid). Thus, early trabeculae consist of a core of calcified cartilage covered by a shell of bone. These are removed through the activity of osteoclasts that appear on the bony shell. In this way, an expanding cavity is formed in the developing shaft. Support is provided by expansion of the periosteal collar, which becomes thicker and longer as the periosteum lays down new bone at the external surface. The process continues as an orderly progression toward **both ends** of the cartilaginous precursor. Several zones of activity can be distinguished in the remaining cartilage. Beginning at the ends furthest from the primary ossification center, these are as follows:

Zone of reserve cartilage. This area consists of typical hyaline cartilage with chondrocytes and their lacunae randomly arranged throughout the matrix.
Zone of proliferation. In this region chondrocytes actively proliferate and as a result chondrocytes become aligned in rows or columns separated only by a small amount of matrix.
Zone of maturation and hypertrophy. Here, cell division stops and chondrocytes mature and enlarge. Lacunae expand at the expense of the intervening matrix and the matrix between adjacent rows of chondrocytes becomes even thinner.
Zone of calcification and cell death. The matrix between and around the rows of chondrocytes becomes calcified and chondrocytes die, degenerate and leave empty lacunae.

The thin regions of matrix between lacunae then break down resulting in irregularly shaped tunnels appearing in the matrix. The extent of this zone can be recognized by careful examination of the matrix, which stains slightly darker than that of the previous zones indicating the extent of calcium diffusion into the matrix.

Zone of ossification. Vascular connective tissue enters the tunnel-like spaces formed in the adjacent zone and provides osteoprogenitor cells that differentiate into osteoblasts. **Osteoblasts** gather on the surface of the calcified cartilage and lay down bone matrix (osteoid). Examine these cells carefully.

Zone of resorption. The calcified cartilage and the bony covering are resorbed due to the action of osteoclasts. In this way the marrow cavity increases in size as the developing bone increases in length. **Osteoclasts** are large multinucleate giant cells with a moderately stained acidophilic cytoplasm. Some may contain as many as 30 nuclei. Individual nuclei show no unusual features and usually are located in the part of the cell furthest from the bone surface. The cell surface adjacent to the bone may show a striated (ruffled) border. Osteoclasts reside in shallow depressions on the surface of bone called **Howship's lacunae**.

Carefully examine and sketch the zones within the cartilage for the details described and then re-examine the periosteal collar.

Simultaneous with these events the periosteal collar increases in thickness and length, extending towards the ends of the developing bone. Its growth continues to provide a splint around the area of weakened cartilage.

Near the time of birth, new centers of ossification (epiphyseal or secondary ossification centers) appear in the epiphyses. Hyaline cartilage of the epiphyses show the same sequence of events as observed in the diaphysis, but growth and subsequent ossification spreads simultaneously in all directions. Ultimately, all the cartilage will be is replaced by bone, except for the free end in the joint cavity, which remains as articular cartilage. Hyaline cartilage also persists as a narrow plate between the diaphysis and epiphysis called the **epiphyseal plate**. Its continued growth permits further elongation of bone. Note that the epiphyseal plate continues to exhibit the various zones associated with endochondral bone formation. When growth in the cartilage plate ceases, it is replaced by bone and further increase in length of the bone is no longer possible. Thus, the rapid growth of a long bone is largely the result of cartilage growth and bone replacement and not growth of bone *per se*. Examine the external surface of the periosteal collar for a layer of osteoblasts and its associated osteoid.

Sketch this region, including its relationship with the surrounding periosteum.

Table 4. Key histologic features used in identifying different types of compact connective tissues.

Type	Arrangement of cells and matrix	Additional features
Hyaline cartilage	Glasslike matrix; lacunae with chondrocytes randomly arranged, slitlike in appearance near perichondrium	Isogenous groups, territorial matrix
Elastic cartilage	Matrix more fibrous in appearance; elastic fibers (need to be stained selectively); lacunae with chondrocytes randomly arranged	Large isogenous groups
Decalcified bone	Lacunae with osteocytes show organization within lamellae of osteons; Haversian canals lined by endosteum contain blood vessels	Tide marks, bone marrow, irregular shape of lacunae
Ground bone	Matrix only arranged into distinct Haversian systems; interstitial and circumferential lamellae	Canaliculi distinct between lacunae
Fibrous cartilage	Dense fibrous appearance with a small amount of ground substance; round cells within lacunae are arranged in short rows between collagenous fibers	Round-shaped chondrocytes
Tendon, ligaments, aponeuroses	Fibroblast nuclei dense staining and elongate, lie in parallel rows between regularly arranged collagen fibers	Lacunae absent
Dermis, capsules of organs, periosteum, perichondrium	Fibroblast nuclei dense and elongate; randomly scattered between dense interwoven, irregular arrangement of collagen fibers	Lacunae absent

Three types of muscle can be distinguished: skeletal, cardiac and smooth.

Learning objectives for muscle tissue:

1. Be able to distinguish between the three types of muscle.

Skeletal muscle

The skeletal muscle cell (fiber) is a giant cell that ranges between 10 and 100 μm in diameter and is extremely variable in length. Skeletal muscle cells are **multinucleated** and may contain several hundred nuclei. All are peripheral in location, evenly spaced immediately beneath the plasmalemma. The nuclei are elongated in the direction of the long axis of the cell. Chromatin tends to be distributed along the nuclear envelope and one or two nucleoli are usually present. The most outstanding structural feature of the skeletal muscle cell is the presence of alternating light and dark **bands** or **cross-striations** that are visible when the cell is viewed in longitudinal section. The **dark bands** are called **A bands** and the **light bands** are called **I bands**. Running transversely through the center of the I band is a narrow dense line, the **Z line**. Myofibrils are elongated, thread-like structures that fill the skeletal muscle cell, compressing the nuclei to a peripheral location. **Myofibrils** are the smallest units of contractile material that can be identified with the light microscope and in transverse section appear as small, solid dots within the muscle cell (fiber). Each myofibril shows the identical banding pattern to that of the whole cell. Indeed, the banding of the skeletal muscle cell results from the bands on the contained myofibrils being in perfect alignment as the plasmalemma of the cell is transparent. Compare the banding seen with the light microscope with that visible in an electron micrograph.

     The interior of the tongue and lip are excellent locations to carefully examine the details of individual skeletal muscle cells. Skeletal muscle is closely associated with connective tissue at all levels of organization. In examining a named muscle, the entire muscle is surrounded by a connective tissue sheath called the **epimysium**. Septa pass from the deep surface of the epimysium to envelop muscle fascicles (groups of muscle cells) as the **perimysium**. A delicate connective tissue wraps each individual muscle cell as an **endomysium**. Although given different names according to its association with different structural units of skeletal muscle, the connective tissue forms a continuum and acts not only to bind the various muscle units together but also functions as a harness and aids in integrating and transmitting the

forces of contraction. It consists of collagenous, reticular and elastic fibers and contains several connective tissue cell types, the most common of which are fibroblasts. The endomysium is delicate and consists primarily of reticular and thin collagen fibers. It contains blood capillaries and small nerve branches. Larger nerves and blood vessels lie within the perimysium.

Sketch and label longitudinal and transverse profiles of skeletal muscle cells. In the transverse profile include its association with the surrounding connective tissue.

Cardiac muscle

Cardiac muscle is associated with the heart and forms the majority of the heart wall or myocardium. Cardiac muscle cells are small cylindrical cells that **branch** and are linked to one another, end to end, by specialized junctions known as **intercalated discs**. The latter appear as darkly stained transverse lines. Each cardiac muscle cell contains one or occasionally two **centrally positioned nuclei**. The same banding pattern witnessed in skeletal muscle occurs in cardiac muscle. Although A bands, I bands and Z lines are visible they are not as conspicuous as those of skeletal muscle. Myofibrils are fewer in number and often grouped into bundles that diverge around nuclei. As a result, regions of cytoplasm appear structureless at each nuclear pole. Examine both longitudinal and transverse profiles of cardiac muscle cells to confirm the position of their nuclei. A web of reticular and fine collagenous fibers is present between cardiac muscle cells and corresponds to an endomysium. Numerous capillaries are present in this layer of connective tissue.

Sketch and label both longitudinal and transverse profiles of cardiac muscle cells. The longitudinal profile should include an intercalated disc. Compare these light microscopic observations with those features seen in electron micrographs of cardiac muscle.

Smooth muscle

Smooth muscle is widely distributed and plays an essential role in the function of organs. It forms the contractile portion of the walls of blood vessels, hollow viscera, such as the digestive, respiratory, urinary and reproductive systems, and is a subcomponent of most other organs.

     Smooth muscle cells are shaped like **elongated spindles** with a **single, central nucleus** occupying the wide portion of the cell midway along its length. The nucleus is elongated in the long axis of the cell. Smooth muscle cells lack the cross-striations observed in the two other forms of muscle.

Smooth muscle cells may be present as small isolated units or may from prominent sheets. In any one sheet of smooth muscle, the cells tend to be **oriented in the same direction** but are offset so that the wide portions of some cells lie adjacent to the tapering ends of neighboring cells. This is most evident in transverse sections, where the outlines of the cells vary in diameter according to where along their lengths the cells were cut. Nuclei are few in this view and present only in muscle cells cut near their largest profiles (centers). A thin connective tissue of fine collagenous, reticular and elastic fibers aids in binding the smooth muscle cells into bundles or sheets. In routine preparations this fine reticuloelastic sheet is almost imperceptible and the field is dominated by profiles of smooth muscle cells.

Examine and sketch the muscle wall of a transversely cut segment of small intestine and note that it consists of two sheets or layers of smooth muscle. The smooth muscle cells in the external layer will be sectioned transversely, those of the adjacent inner layer will be cut parallel to their long axis. Examine the smooth muscle cells carefully at higher magnifications and note the position of their nuclei.

Next, examine the wall of any named artery for its smooth muscle layer, which occupies the center of the vessel wall. What is the orientation of cells within this smooth muscle layer? How can smooth muscle cells be differentiated from adjacent fibroblasts?

Table 5. Key histologic features that distinguish muscle types.				
Type	**Cell shape**	**Nuclei**	**Striations**	**Other features**
Skeletal	Long cylinders	Peripheral, multiple	Present	Endomysium, perimysium
Cardiac	Short branching, anastomosing cylinders	Central, usually single, occasional double	Present	Intercalated discs
Smooth	Small spindles	Central, single	Absent	Cells packed tightly together, occurs in sheets, layers or bundles with nuclei oriented in the same direction

Neurons (nerve cells)

It should be emphasized that the majority of cell bodies (perikarya) of neurons are found in the gray matter of the central nervous system (CNS). Aggregates of perikarya occur in the gray matter of the CNS, which act as distinct functional units called **nuclei**. Similar collections of individual nerve cell bodies are located outside the CNS and these are called **ganglia**. Thus, the majority of nerve tissue (the nerves) seen in the peripheral nervous system are the processes of nerve cells and do not contain the soma or cell body.

Learning objectives for nerve tissue:

1. Be able to find, identify and classify neurons in the central and peripheral nervous system.
2. Be able to identify sections of peripheral nerve in other tissues.
3. Be able to locate and identify encapsulated sensory nerve endings as well as motor end plates.
4. Be able to compare and contrast the morphology of dorsal root (cranio-spinal) and autonomic chain ganglia.
5. Be able to find and identify the various forms of neuroglia.
6. Be able to differentiate between a section of spinal cord, cerebellar cortex and cerebral cortex and identify the major subcomponents of each.

Examine a transverse section of spinal cord with the low-power objective. Note that it is divided into an outer, limiting layer of **white matter** and a central, butterfly-shaped region of **gray matter**. A small central canal lies at the center of the spinal cord. The gray matter is subdivided into two smaller dorsal horns and two larger ventral horns. Examine the ventral gray matter for **large multipolar neurons, which are obvious,** even under low power. These neurons are large and complex in shape and consist of a cell body, the **perikaryon**, and several cytoplasmic processes. The majority of the processes are dendrites as each neuron has but a single axon conducting impulses away from the perikaryon. Examine a perikaryon and identify the large, round euchromatic **nucleus** as well as a dense-staining central **nucleolus**. Special staining methods, such as pyridine silver, can be used to demonstrate bundles of **neurofibrils** which from an anastomosing network around the nucleus and extend into the dendrites and axon. Likewise, dyes such as cresyl violet or toluidine blue can be used to demonstrate basophilic masses, **chromophilic (Nissl) substance**, within the cytoplasm of the perikaryon

and dendrites. Nissl substance is absent from the **axon** and the **axon hillock**, the region of the perikaryon from which the axon originates. The motor neurons of the ventral gray matter are a classic example of large **multipolar** neurons. Note that a nucleus is not observed in each neuron. Why is this?

Sketch and label several multipolar neurons.

For an example of **pseudounipolar** neurons, examine a preparation of **spinal ganglion**. Observe that the ganglion is enveloped by a connective tissue capsule and may contain perikarya of only a few hundred neurons or several thousand. A delicate network of collagenous and reticular fibers, accompanied by small blood vessels, extends between individual neurons and, together with bundles of nerve processes, often separates the perikarya into groups. The perikarya are large (15 - 100 μm in diameter), spherical in shape and exhibit distinct central, round nuclei and nucleoli. Two distinct capsules envelop the perikarya. The **inner capsule** consists of a single layer of cuboidal supporting cells, known as **satellite cells**. An **outer capsule** of delicate, vascular connective tissue lies immediately outside the basement membrane of the satellite cells. A single nerve process is associated with the pseudounipolar neuron, which may become highly convoluted. This nerve process then divides: one branch, a **functional axon**, passes into the central nervous system; the other, a **functional dendrite**, passes to a receptor organ. The perikarya of these pseudounipolar neurons <u>do not</u> receive synapses from other neurons.

In contrast, **autonomic ganglia** consist of **multipolar neurons** of various sizes and shapes and receive considerable synaptic input from other neurons. Perikarya range between 15 and 60 μm in diameter and the large round nucleus often lies eccentrically placed within the cell. Binucleate cells are not an uncommon observation. Gold-brown granules (lipofuscin granules) are a more frequent observation within perikarya of autonomic ganglia than in craniospinal ganglia. Perikarya of larger sympathetic chain ganglia may show partial encapsulation by satellite cells, but such a capsule may be absent around ganglia in the walls of the viscera. Examine an autonomic ganglion (myenteric plexus) in the wall of the small intestine. It can be found in the seam of connective tissue separating the circular and longitudinal layers of smooth muscle (muscularis externa) forming the gut wall.

Examples of **bipolar neurons**, neurons with a single dendrite and axon usually located at opposite poles of the perikaryon, can be found in the cochlear and vestibular ganglia of the inner ear as well as in the retina.

Compare and contrast a labeled sketch of neurons (the perikarya) found within a spinal ganglion and an autonomic ganglion.

Peripheral nerves

Examine both transverse and longitudinal sections of an isolated, named peripheral nerve if possible. These are mixed nerves consisting of sensory (afferent) and motor (efferent) nerve fibers that may be myelinated or unmyelinated. The sheath of connective tissue surrounding a peripheral nerve is called the **epineurium**. It unites several bundles of nerve fibers or fascicles into a single unit, the peripheral nerve. The epineurium consists of longitudinally oriented collagen fibers and fibroblasts organized to form a spiral of large pitch about the long axis of the nerve. The epineurium also contains small blood vessels and scattered fat cells. Each **fascicle** of nerve fibers is bounded by concentric layers of flattened, fibroblast-like cells that form a thin, dense sheath called the **perineurium**. Reticular fibers, delicate collagen fibers, fibroblasts and macrophages occur between individual nerve fibers within each fascicle and form the **endoneurium**. Networks of small capillaries can be found within the endoneurium.

Peripheral nerve fibers

A nerve fiber is defined as an **axon (axis cylinder)** and a surrounding sheath of **Schwann cells**. Schwann cells are thin, attenuated cells with flattened, elongate nuclei located near the center of the cell. The nucleoplasm is often finely stippled and plumper in appearance than the thin, densely stained nuclear profiles of fibroblasts in the adjacent endoneurium. Schwann cells may or may not be associated with a lipoprotein material called **myelin** in smaller nerve fibers. Thus, peripheral nerve fibers may be classified as being either myelinated or unmyelinated. In both myelinated and unmyelinated nerve fibers, Schwann cells invest the axis cylinders from near their beginnings almost to their terminations and form the **neurilemma**. In myelinated nerve fibers, the neurilemmal and myelin sheaths are interrupted by small gaps at regular intervals along the course of a nerve fiber and are called the **nodes of Ranvier**. The region between two consecutive nodes of Ranvier constitutes one **internode** or **internodal segment**. The internode represents the area occupied by a single Schwann cell. Examine the longitudinal profile of a peripheral nerve for both nodes of Ranvier and internodal segments. These are easily seen in frozen sections that have been stained with osmic acid (osmium) to demonstrate myelin sheaths, which appear as a solid black material. In routinely prepared sections stained with H&E, the myelin sheath may appear as an empty space due to the removal of lipid or as a network of residual protein called **neurokeratin**. This is simply a residue of myelin following processing. Nodes of Ranvier appear as regions where the thin neurilemma approaches the axis cylinder on either side. The myelin sheath between the neurilemma and the axis cylinder may be empty or contain neurokeratin. Identify several Schwann cell nuclei oriented with their elongated profiles lying parallel to the long axis of the nerve fibers. Clearly distinguish Schwann cell nuclei from adjacent fibroblast nuclei of the endoneurium, which are more slender and stain more intensely. Examine several nerve fibers that have been cut transversely and identify the central axis cylinder, the myelin space and the limiting neurilemma. Nuclear profiles of Schwann cells can, on occasion, be observed coursing around the myelin space. Note again the relationship of the endoneurium between nerve fibers.

Compare labeled sketches of longitudinal and transverse sections of large peripheral nerves.

Nerve tissue

Having completed a study of an isolated peripheral nerve, examine a section of lip or tongue and identify peripheral nerves of smaller caliber coursing in the tissue near the skeletal muscle. Look at both longitudinal and transverse profiles. Small peripheral nerves can be differentiated from surrounding connective tissue by examining the latter for small round or cylindrical units bounded by perineurium that are lighter staining and show a structural organization. An additional feature characteristic of peripheral nerves is that they often present a wavy or undulating course through the surrounding connective tissue. The latter also stains more intensely than does nerve tissue. Once located, examine the peripheral nerve at increased magnification and note that the Schwann cell nuclei are all oriented in the same direction and that there are more nuclei per unit area as compared to the fewer, randomly organized fibroblast nuclei of the surrounding connective tissue. Identify the myelin sheath (or its space), axis cylinders and nodes of Ranvier in a small peripheral nerve coursing through the connective tissue.

Make a sketch of nerves coursing among other tissues.

Nerve endings

The most common nerve endings seen in routine preparations are the encapsulated sensory nerve endings. **Meissner's corpuscles** are commonly found in the connective tissue of the dermal papillae in the digits. Note the spiral architecture of the connective tissue forming the capsule. Examine the much larger **lamellated corpuscles of Vater-Pacini.** These are often found in the deep dermis of the skin or in the pancreas. These large corpuscles can easily be found by scanning with the low-power objective. Their architecture appears much like that of an onion that has been divided in half. The pale nerve ending can often be visualized near the center of this structure. If special preparations are available, the **motor end plates** of skeletal muscle should be examined. The latter generally are not easily seen in routine H&E preparations. Synaptic endings of axons can be found in good, specially stained preparations. They usually occur as small swellings at the tips of axon branches and are called **terminal boutons**. These can be observed in pyridine silver preparations of the spinal cord. Carefully examine the external surface of the large multipolar neurons in the ventral gray matter of the spinal cord under oil emersion for these structures.

Sketch and compare as many of the nerve endings as possible.

Neuroglia

Neuroglia are generally smaller than neurons and can be identified by their small, round nuclei which are scattered among neurons and their processes in the CNS. Two forms of neuroglia, astrocytes and oligodendrocytes, are often collectively referred to as macroglia. The cytoplasmic extent of these cells can be demonstrated only with special staining techniques. The astrocytes can be divided into protoplasmic and fibrous types dependent on their morphology and position within the CNS. **Protoplasmic astrocytes** are characterized by numerous, thick branching processes and are found mainly in the gray matter. **Fibrous astrocytes** are distinguished by long, thin, generally unbranched processes and occur mainly in the white matter. The processes of both often expand to form end feet that are associated with the walls of blood vessels or aligned along the internal surface of the pia mater. **Oligodendrocytes** are smaller cells with fewer processes and more deeply stained, round nuclei. **Microglia** (macrophages of the CNS) also are small cells with extensive ramifying processes and exhibit a characteristic dendritic phenotype suggestive of antigen-presenting cells. **Ependymal cells** are a form of glia that line the central canal of the spinal cord and the ventricles of the brain. They consist of a single layer of closely packed cells that vary in shape from cuboidal to columnar. The ependyma also forms, in areas where it is in direct contact with and covers a highly vascular region of the pia mater called the tela choroidea, the choroid plexus. The choroid plexus is involved in the production of cerebrospinal fluid. Together, the closely packed columnar ependymal cells and the tela choroidea (a delicate vascularized connective tissue) form the **choroid plexus**.

Ganglia

Compare and contrast a section of **dorsal root ganglion** with that of an **autonomic chain ganglion**. Note the more complete encapsulation of individual nerve cell bodies in the dorsal root ganglion. Recall that these are large **pseudounipolar neurons** with centrally positioned nuclei. The perikarya often appear to be organized and separated into groups by bundles of nerve fibers. In contrast, the perikarya from autonomic ganglia generally are smaller, often exhibit eccentric nuclei and the cytoplasm often contains an abundance of pigment (lipofuscin) granules. Note the irregular outline of individual perikarya. This is due to numerous processes associated with these **multipolar neurons**.

Make a sketch comparing a dorsal root ganglion with an autonomic chain ganglion.

Central nervous system

Spinal cord

The spinal cord is subdivided into a central butterfly-shaped region of gray matter and a surrounding layer of white matter. **Gray matter** is arranged into two dorsal and two ventral horns and consists mainly of perikarya of neurons, their dendrites and neuroglial cells. The multipolar neurons in the ventral horns are the largest cells in the spinal cord. In the thoracic and upper lumbar regions of the spinal cord, small multipolar neurons form an **intermediolateral horn** that provides preganglionic sympathetic fibers for the autonomic nervous system. The **central canal** lies in the center of the cross bar of the butterfly-shaped gray matter and is lined by ependyma. The **white matter** consists mainly of myelinated axons. It is subdivided into anterior, lateral, and posterior funiculi by the dorsal and ventral horns of the gray matter.

Make a sketch of an entire transverse section of spinal cord and label its subcomponents.

Brain

The cerebellar and cerebral hemispheres differ from the spinal cord in that the gray matter is located at the periphery. The white matter lies centrally. Thus, both regions of the brain consist of an outer cortex of gray matter and a subcortical area of white matter.

Cerebellar cortex

The cerebellar cortex consists of three layers: an outer molecular layer, a middle Purkinje cell layer and an inner granule layer. The **molecular layer** consists primarily of unmyelinated axons running parallel to the cortical surface and exhibits only a few nerve cells. It also contains large dendrites extending from Purkinje cells in the underlying layer. The small scattered neurons in the superficial portion of this layer are called **stellate cells**.

The **Purkinje cell layer** is formed by the perikarya of the **Purkinje cells**. This layer consists of very large, pear-shaped perikarya aligned in a single row. The Purkinje cell is characterized by large branching dendrites that extend into and lie in the molecular layer. These large dendritic trees occupy a narrow three-dimensional plane, similar to fan coral, and are so arranged that each dendritic tree lies parallel to its neighbor. In H&E preparations only the base of the dendritic tree can be visualized. It is only with special staining (Golgi silver impregnation stain) that the full extent of this large dendritic tree can be appreciated. The **granule cell layer** consists of numerous closely packed, small neurons. They have small round nuclei with coarse chromatin patterns and only a scant amount of cytoplasm. They form a darkly stained layer, several cells deep, immediately deep to the Purkinje cell layer.

Draw and label a sketch of a region from the cerebellar cortex.

Cerebral cortex

The cerebral cortex is 1.5 - 4.0 mm thick and in all but a few regions is characterized by a laminated appearance. The neuronal perikarya of the cerebral cortex generally are organized into **five indistinct layers**. Beginning at the periphery the cerebral cortex can be subdivided into the following:

1. molecular layer;
2. external granular layer;
3. external pyramidal layer;
4. internal granular layer;
5. internal pyramidal layer; and
6. multiform layer.

The molecular layer is primarily a cell-free zone just beneath the cortical surface. Neurons of similar morphology tend to occupy the same layers in the cerebral cortex. For convenience these neurons are placed in two major groups: pyramidal cells and non-pyramidal cells. Perikarya of **pyramidal cells** are pyramidal in shape and have a large apical dendrite, usually oriented toward the surface of the cerebral cortex and entering the overlying layers. They are found in layers 2,3,5 and to a lesser degree in layer 6. Very large pyramidal neurons called **Betz cells** are present in layer 5 of the frontal lobe. In routine H&E preparations it is only the shape of the perikaryon and the base of the apical dendrite that are seen. The extent of the dendrites can be traced by using special silver-staining techniques (Golgi stain) as was the case for examining the dendritic tree of Purkinje cells in the cerebellum. **Non-pyramidal cells** lack the large apical dendrite and the pyramidal-shaped perikarya. They are found in all layers of the cerebral cortex but are concentrated in layer 4 (the internal granular layer).

Make a labeled sketch of a section through the cerebral cortex. Compare this sketch with the one made of the cerebellar cortex.

Table 6. Key histologic features of primary cell types of nerve tissue.

Location of Perikarya	Morphology	Other features
Neurons of the peripheral nervous system		
Cranial and spinal ganglia	Large, round, pseudounipolar; distinct central nucleus with nucleolus	Each perikaryon surrounded by satellite cells
Sympathetic chain ganglia, parasympathetic ganglia in walls of organs	Size variable, stellate; multipolar; nucleus often eccentric; lipofuscin granules common	Axons usually unmyelinated
Neurons of the central nervous system		
Gray matter of spinal cord	Multipolar, stellate, size variable; distinct nuclei and nucleoli	Perikarya occur in groups or columns
Gray matter of cerebral cortex	Multipolar, pyramidal with large apical dendrite; stellate cells with round nuclei; lack apical dendrite	Perikarya organized into 5 indistinct layers
Gray matter of cerebellar cortex	Multipolar, Purkinje cell and small neurons of granule layer characteristic	Organized into 3 distinct layers
Glia of the peripheral nervous system		
Schwann cells	Flattened, elongated; heterochromatic nucleus in center of cell	Envelope axon to form neurilemmal sheath; form myelin in peripheral nervous system
Satellite cells (amphicytes)	Single layer of low cuboidal cells; nuclei heterochromatic, cytoplasm clear and indistinct	Surround neuronal perikarya; continuous with neurilemma
Glia of the central nervous system		
Fibrous astrocytes	Pale-staining ovoid or spherical nucleus, sparse heterochromatin; long, thin , unbranched processes	Primarily in white matter
Protoplasmic astrocytes	Pale-staining ovoid or spherical nucleus, sparse heterochromatin; short, thick, branching processes	Primarily in gray matter
Interfascicular oligodendrocytes	Small cell (6-8 μm); ovoid or spherical, deeply stained nuclei; few processes	Envelope axons of white matter; form myelin in central nervous system
Perineuronal oligodendrocytes	Same as above	Gray matter; closely associated with perikarya of neurons
Ependyma	Simple cuboidal to columnar	Line central canal of spinal cord; ventricles of brain

CHAPTER 7. PERIPHERAL BLOOD AND BONE MARROW

Blood

The formed elements of blood include erythrocytes, platelets and leukocytes.

Learning objectives for peripheral blood:

1. Be able to distinguish the formed elements (both normal and recognize abnormal forms if present) in a smear of normal peripheral blood.

Erythrocytes

The erythrocyte is anucleate and appears as a biconcave disc. Erythrocytes are uniformly acidophilic and devoid of any internal structure. In smears they average 7.6 μm in diameter, being slightly smaller in tissue sections (6.5-7.0 μm) and in fresh blood are slightly larger (8.0 μm). The thickness of the erythrocyte is about 2.0 μm. Most erythrocytes stain orange-red but a few, when stained with brilliant cresyl blue or new methylene blue dye, exhibit a central basophilic network. These are immature erythrocytes called **reticulocytes**. Reticulocytes make up only 1-2% of the erythrocytes in normal peripheral blood.

Abnormalities of erythrocytes

Departures from normal size, shape or staining properties can be important indicators of disease. Some of these abnormalities may be found in healthy individuals also but to a lesser degree. **Anisocytosis** refers to abnormal variations in size. **Macrocytes** are erythrocytes larger than normal; **microcytes** smaller than normal. Irregularity of shape is referred to as **poikilocytosis**. Under a variety of conditions, erythrocytes *in vitro* may become shrunken and exhibit numerous projections. Such cells are called **echinocytes** and are said to be **crenated.** Severe changes in shape occur during sickling of erythrocytes in sickle cell anemia. In this condition, erythrocytes may appear as holly leaves, crescents or tubes. **Hypochromia** refers to erythrocytes that stain weakly due to a decrease in hemoglobin. Staining may consist of only a narrow peripheral band, or in erythrocytes thinner than normal (leptocytes) stain as *target cells* in which the staining occurs as a central disk and an external band separated by an unstained zone. *Siderocytes* are erythrocytes that contain clusters of small granules that react positively for iron. Examine several erythrocytes in a smear of peripheral blood for any of these abnormalities.

Platelets

Platelets are small, anucleate round bodies 2-4 μm in diameter and the second most numerous of the formed elements in blood. Platelets are not true cells but fragments of cytoplasm derived from megakaryocytes in the bone marrow. In stained blood smears, platelets exhibit a darker staining **granulomere** (chromomere) in the central region and a surrounding pale, granule-free **hyalomere**. Because of their friable nature, tiny light blue fragments of platelets are the most common observation scattered between erythrocytes. Look for, and identify, several platelet fragments and attempt to locate an intact platelet.

Leukocytes

Leukocytes (white blood cells) are the only true cells of peripheral blood and have nuclei. Leukocytes can be classed as polymorphonuclear or mononuclear according to the shape of the nucleus or granular or agranular on the basis of cytoplasmic granulation. Granular leukocytes and polymorphonuclear leukocytes denote the same class of cell. Likewise, the terms agranular and mononuclear leukocytes indicate the same class of cell.

Polymorphonuclear (granular) leukocytes

Neutrophil leukocytes (polys) vary from 12 to 15 μm in diameter and are characterized by a nucleus that consists of **three to five nuclear lobes** connected by thin **nuclear filaments**. The nucleus stains deeply and the chromatin is aggregated into clumps that form a patchy network. Nucleoli are absent. Nuclear appendages, in the shape of hooks, racquets, clubs or drumsticks, may be present. Of these, only the **drumstick** is significant and represents female sex chromatin. It occurs on a terminal nuclear lobe in about 2-3% of neutrophils from women. Examine several neutrophils for this appendage. Drumsticks are not observed in neutrophils of men. The fine cytoplasmic granules often take on a light pinkish hue or remain relatively unstained. Neutrophils form 50 - 70% of the circulating leukocytes and therefore are the most commonly observed leukocyte.

     Eosinophil leukocytes are about the same size as neutrophils and also show nuclear lobulation. Although many have a bilobed nucleus, eosinophils with three or four nuclear lobes are not uncommon. The distinctive feature of eosinophils is the presence of closely packed, uniform **granules** in the cytoplasm that **stain a brilliant red or orange-red**.

Eosinophils make up about 3% of the circulating leukocytes. Identify a bilobed eosinophil that presents the classical "spectacled" appearance.

Basophil leukocytes are slightly smaller than neutrophils and measure 10-12 μm in blood smears. Nuclear lobes are less distinct than those of either the neutrophil or eosinophil. Nuclei with more than two or three lobes are rare. The nuclear filaments between lobes are short and broad and rarely form the thread-like structures observed in neutrophils. The chromatin is relatively homogeneous and less intensely stained than in the other two granulocytes. Nucleoli are absent. The cytoplasm of basophils contains **prominent granules** that stain a **deep violet** with standard blood stains. Well-preserved granules are spherical and uniform, however, being soluble in water or glycerin, may be partially extracted. Thus, some granules may appear empty or irregular in size and shape in fixed preparations. They are scattered unevenly in the cytoplasm and often overlie the nucleus. Some may lie near the plasma membrane, bulge outward and give the perimeter of the cell a scalloped appearance. Granules are not as numerous nor as densely packed as granules of eosinophil leukocytes. Basophils make up about 0.5% of the total leukocytes and therefore are the most difficult to find and study.

Mononuclear (agranular) leukocytes

Lymphocytes comprise a family of cells differing in size, life span and functions.

Small lymphocytes are the most common type. They have a diameter of 6 - 8 μm and appear as little more than a nucleus enveloped by a thin rim of transparent blue cytoplasm. On one side of the cell, the cytoplasm may be slightly expanded. The nucleus may be indented slightly, is heterochromatic and stains deeply. Lymphocytes are the predominant agranulocyte and in the adult account for 20 - 35% of the circulating leukocytes. Although morphologically indistinguishable by ordinary stains, small lymphocytes are a mixture of two major classes: B and T lymphocytes. Larger lymphocytes, 10 - 14 μm in diameter, are also present in peripheral blood but in small numbers. The cytoplasm of these cells is more abundant than that of the small lymphocyte.

Monocytes are the second type of mononuclear leukocyte normally found in peripheral blood. They vary in size from 12 - 20 μm in diameter and contain a fairly large nucleus that may be either rounded, kidney-shaped or horseshoe shaped. The chromatin is more loosely dispersed than in lymphocytes and stains less densely. Two or three nucleoli may be seen. The gray-blue cytoplasm is abundant and has a "ground glass" or "dusty" appearance. Monocytes form 3 - 8% of the circulating leukocytes.

Note: If difficulty is encountered finding the various leukocytes, examine those areas near the edge of the coverslip and in particular the end of the slide furthest from where the original drop of blood was placed. It must be remembered that this preparation is a **blood smear**. In this case a drop of blood is placed at one end and then with the aid of another slide smeared or pulled toward the opposite end of the slide. As leukocytes are the lightest formed elements in blood they tend to flow to the edges of the slide and many are dragged to the opposite end of the slide.

Make a composite sketch of a smear of peripheral blood illustrating all of the formed elements.

Table 7. Key cytologic features that distinguish the formed elements found in peripheral blood.

Cell	Diameter (μm)	Cytoplasm	Nucleus	Nucleolus
Erythrocytes	7.6	Biconcave disc, eosinophilic	No	No
Platelets	2.0-4.0	Chromomere light blue, hyalomere pale	No	No
Neutrophils	10-15	Numerous fine granules, lilac color	2-4 dense lobes connected by a fine nuclear filament	No
Eosinophils	10-14	Numerous coarse, red-orange granules	2 dense lobes connected by nuclear filament usual, 3-5 lobes may occur	No
Basophils	10-12	Round, blue-black granules	Less distinct lobulation, broad nuclear filament	No
Small lymphocytes	6-8	Thin, blue rim	Round, dark staining	Yes
Large lymphocytes	10-14	Abundant, light transparent blue	Round, lighter staining than small form	Yes
Monocytes	12-20	Abundant, bluish gray, opaque in appearance	Large, kidney or horseshoe shape	Yes

Hemopoietic tissue

Formed elements of the blood are **not self-replicating** and their numbers in the circulation are maintained by continuous replacement from specialized blood-forming (**hemopoietic**) tissues **outside** the vascular system. In the adult these consist of the bone marrow, spleen, lymph nodes and the thymus.

Bone marrow

Bone marrow is a very cellular connective tissue that fills the marrow cavity of bone and may have a red or yellow color. **Yellow (fatty) marrow** is inactive and its principal cellular components are fat cells. **Red marrow** is actively engaged in the production of blood cells and is the hemopoietic marrow. On the basis of its fiber content, bone marrow can be classed as a **reticular connective tissue**. A loose network of reticular fibers and associated reticular cells (specialized fibroblasts laying down and maintaining reticular fibers) fills the marrow cavities of bone and provides the supporting framework for hemopoietic cells. Reticular cells have large, elongate pale-staining nuclei and an irregular light-staining cytoplasm. **Sinusoids** (venous sinuses) are thin-walled vessels 15 - 100 μm in diameter that form an extensive network throughout the bone marrow. They are lined by thin, flattened endothelial cells. The actual hemopoietic

elements form irregular cords of cells between the sinusoids **outside** the vascular compartment. In sections of bone marrow some ordering of the blood-forming cells can be seen. Erythrocytes develop as small islets close to the sinusoids, with some ordering of cells within a given cluster. The most mature cells occupy the outer rim of the cluster. Developing granulocytes form islets that tend to be at some distance from the sinusoids. It is important to realize that **bone marrow is most often examined in smears** following aspiration of marrow from bone. The smear is made the same way as a smear of peripheral blood. Thus, all relationships are destroyed and a mixture of supporting elements and hemopoietic cells results. It is this mixture of randomly arranged cells that must be dealt with in a marrow smear.

Learning objectives for a bone marrow smear:

1. Be able to distinguish the various stages of maturation associated with erythropoiesis and understand what the morphological changes signify during the transformation to a mature erythrocyte.
2. Be able to distinguish the various stages of maturation associated with granulocytopoiesis and understand what the morphological changes signify during the transformation of each to the mature granulocytes.
3. Be able to identify megakaryocytes and platelets and have an understanding of thrombocytopoiesis.

4. Be able to identify monocytes, lymphocytes and plasma cells and have a basic understanding of the interrelationships of these cells.

Development of erythrocytes

Erythropoiesis is the process of erythrocyte production. During this transformation, the developing erythrocytes undergo progressive changes that involve both the nucleus and the cytoplasm. The cell progressively becomes smaller, the cytoplasm changes color from deep blue to pink as it accumulates hemoglobin and looses organelles and the nucleus shrinks and condenses until it ultimately is lost from the cell. Although the process is a continuous one, at several points the cells show distinctive, recognizable features. These morphological stages are as follows:

The **proerythroblast** is the earliest recognizable precursor of the erythrocyte cell line. It is relatively large with a diameter of 15 - 25 μm. The **non-granular, basophilic cytoplasm** often stains unevenly exhibiting regions that are poorly stained especially in a zone close to the nucleus. The **round, central nucleus** occupies nearly three-quarters of the cell and its chromatin is **finely** and **uniformly stippled** in appearance. **Two** or **more nucleoli** are usually present and may be prominent. **Note:** As cells of a smear are whole cells rather than sections through cells, the nucleoli often appear as clear or light vacuoles in the nucleoplasm.

The **basophilic erythroblast** generally is smaller than the proerythroblast, ranging between 12 and 16 μm in diameter. The round, central nucleus continues to occupy a large part of the cell, but the chromatin is more coarsely clumped and deeply stained. Nucleoli generally are absent. The cytoplasm stains evenly and deeply basophilic, generally more so than that of the proerythroblast.

The size of the **polychromatophilic erythroblast** varies considerably (between 10 and 15 μm) but is usually less than that of the basophilic erythroblast. This stage is divided into early and late stages on the basis of their size and on the intensity of the cytoplasmic basophilia. The round, central nucleus occupies a smaller portion of the cell and shows a more dense chromatin pattern with scattered coarse clumps of chromatin. Nucleoli are absent. The cytoplasmic staining varies from bluish gray in early polychromatophilic erythroblasts to slate gray in late stages.

The cytoplasm of **acidophilic erythroblasts (normoblasts)** is almost completely hemoglobinized and stains with a distinctive eosinophilic tint. The nucleus is small, densely stained and pyknotic. It often occupies an eccentric location in the cell. The normoblast ranges from 8 to10 μm in diameter.

After loss of the nucleus, the immature erythrocyte is held in the marrow for 2 - 3 days until fully mature. They have about a 20% larger volume than normal mature erythrocytes and contain a few ribosomes. Only a few of these cells (less than 2%) contain sufficient amounts to impart color to the cytoplasm. These cells have a grayish tint instead of the clear pink of the more mature forms and sometimes are referred to as **polychromatophilic erythrocytes** or **reticulocytes**.

Development of polymorphonuclear (granular) leukocytes

Granulocytopoiesis is the maturational process that leads to the production of mature granular leukocytes. During this process the cells accumulate granules and the nucleus becomes flattened and indented, finally assuming the lobulated form of the adult cell. As with erythrocyte formation, the maturational changes observed during granulocyte formation are a continuum and cells of intermediate morphology are found.

Myeloblasts are the first recognizable precursors of granular leukocytes and are present in the bone marrow only in low numbers. They are relatively small cells, ranging between 10 and 13 μm in diameter. A rounded or oval nucleus occupies much of the cell, stains lightly and has a somewhat vesicular appearance. Multiple nucleoli are present. The cytoplasm is scant, basophilic and lacks granules.

The **promyelocyte** is larger than the myeloblast and measures 15 - 20 μm in diameter. The nucleus may be flattened slightly, show a small indentation or retain a round shape. The chromatin is lightly stained and dispersed. Multiple nucleoli are still present. The lightly basophilic cytoplasm contains scattered **red-purple azurophil granules**, which increase in number as the promyelocyte develops.

The three distinct lines (neutrophil, eosinophil, basophil) of granulocyte appear at the myelocyte stage with the appearance of **specific granules**. **Myelocytes** are smaller than promyelocytes measuring 12-18 μm in diameter. The nucleus is often eccentric, round or indented and the chromatin more condensed. **Neutrophilic, eosinophilic** and **basophilic myelocytes** can be identified by the presence of their specific granules.

Metamyelocytes show most of the cytoplasmic features of the myelocyte. In metamyelocytes the nucleus is deeply indented to form a horseshoe or kidney shape and the chromatin forms a dense network with several masses of well-defined chromatin. **Neutrophil, eosinophil** and **basophil metamyelocytes** can be identified. They measure 12 - 16 μm in diameter.

Band forms have the same general morphology as the mature granulocytes except the nucleus is in the form of a variously curved, twisted band or ribbon. The nucleus may show signs of segmentation but definite nuclear lobes and filaments have yet to form. The chromatin is coarse and stains more intensely than earlier stages. **Neutrophil, eosinophil** and **basophil bands** measure between 10 and 14 μm in diameter. The maturational process is complete with the appearance of distinct nuclear filaments and lobes.

Megakaryocytes and platelets

Thrombocytopoiesis refers to the formation of **platelets**. Platelets form from giant cells called **megakaryocytes** that measure 100 μm or more in diameter. The megakaryocyte nucleus is large, convoluted and consists of multiple irregular lobes of variable size interconnected by constricted regions. The chromatin forms a coarse pattern and stains deeply. The cytoplasm is abundant and often has blunt pseudopods extending from the surface. The cytoplasm appears homogeneous and contains azurophilic granules. Platelets are formed by segmentation of the megakaryocyte cytoplasm. Masses of light blue-staining platelets are often found scattered within a bone marrow smear and on occasion can be observed forming at the peripheral edge of the megakaryocyte cytoplasm. **Hint:** These large cells can be found most easily and quickly by scanning the marrow preparation with the low-power objective.

Development of mononuclear (agranular) leukocytes

Monocytes of bone marrow form from promonocytes, which are rare and difficult to distinguish. They range from 8 to 15 μm in diameter and exhibit a large, round to oval nucleus with evenly dispersed chromatin. Several nucleoli are a common feature. Cytoplasm is abundant and contains a few scattered azurophilic granules. Mature monocytes of the bone marrow closely resemble those of peripheral blood.

Lymphocytes also will be encountered in a smear of bone marrow and appear similar to those in peripheral blood. They can be differentiated from other cells found in the bone marrow by noting the clear, transparent blue-staining nature of the narrow rim of surrounding cytoplasm. Compare the light blue cytoplasm observed in various lymphocytes with that associated with cells in the developing erythrocyte series. Note the differences in the texture of the cytoplasm: that associated with developing erythrocytes appears chalky, as if colored using a crayon; in contrast, cytoplasm of lymphocytes appears clear and transparent, as if colored using watercolors. Note, as well, differences in the nuclear profile. Nuclear profiles of erythroid cells of similar size as lymphocytes will exhibit a clumped chromatin pattern or a very dense nucleoplasm. Lymphocyte nuclei are slightly indented on one side and lighter staining. Nucleoli are also present. **Note:** Refer to the thymus in Chapter 9 as a location to observe and examine large, medium and small lymphocytes. In this case, the small lymphocyte is generally regarded as the more mature form.

Plasma cells also will be observed in bone marrow. These are similar in appearance to those examined in general connective tissue but will appear much larger in size. This is because the preparation is a smear and the plasma cell is spread due to the smearing process. Be aware that the plasma cells examined previously were sectioned plasma cells and therefore appear smaller. Note the very large negative Golgi image, which can be an important clue in its identification. Note also the eccentric position of the nucleus and the large amount of coarse basophilic cytoplasm.

Make a composite sketch of the classic stages observed in the formation of erythrocytes. Note in particular the changes in size, staining of the cytoplasm and the character of the nucleus. Make an addition composite sketch illustrating the changes that occur during formation of the granular leukocyte series. Note the type and appearance of granules present as well as the status of the nucleus at each classic stage. Compare cells from both series. Illustrate the relationship between megakaryocytes and platelet formation.

Reflection

When examining either the erythrocytic or granulocytic cell lines, the morphology observed at each stage should be correlated with the maturational events that ultimately result in the mature cell. For example: nucleoli are a prominent feature of the proerythroblast, the stage of actively involved in the production of ribosomal RNA. Following ribosomal production, nucleoli are lost and the nucleus itself condenses, becomes pyknotic and is extruded in later stages. Likewise, as ribosomal RNA enters the cytoplasm and free ribosomes and polyribosomes becomes a prominent feature of the basophilic erythroblast, the cytoplasm stains increasingly basophilic (royal blue). In later stages the cytoplasm becomes increasingly acidophilic (red-orange) due to an increase in the amount of hemoglobin and a simultaneous loss of ribosomal RNA.

A similar sequence of events occurs in granulocytes. Promyelocytes exhibit multiple nucleoli involved in the production of ribosomal RNA essential for the synthesis of specific granules that appear at the myelocyte stage. Ultrastructurally, these cells show abundant granular endoplasmic reticulum and a well developed Golgi complex, features essential for the production of granules. Following the appearance of specific granules, nucleoli disappear, the eccentric nucleus indents, condenses and eventually forms a narrow ribbon-like structure before segmenting into lobes and filaments characteristic of the adult form.

Cells	Diameter (μm)	Cytoplasm	Nucleus	Nucleolus
Table 8. Key cytologic features of bone marrow hemopoietic cells.				
Myeloblast	10-13	Light blue, transparent, lacks granules	Round or oval with pale staining, fine vesicular chromatin	Yes
Promyelocyte	15-22	Light blue, transparent, scattered azurophil granules	Round or oval, may have slight indent; fine, lightly staining, dispersed chromatin	Yes
Myelocyte	12-18	Light blue, obscured by granules; specific granules (neutrophil, eosinophil, basophil) are now present	Round or oval, often with slight indent, chromatin deeply stained and condensed	No
Metamyelocyte	12-16	Light blue, completely obscured by specific granules, a few azurophil granules present	Horseshoe- or kidney-shaped; coarse masses of deeply stained chromatin	No
Band	10-14	Filled with specific granules; a few azurophil granules present	Ribbon-like, twisted or coiled, no filaments; coarse, deeply stained chromatin	No
Megakaryocyte	50-80	Light blue, transparent; scattered azurophil granules	Large, convoluted, irregular; stains deeply; coarsely patterned chromatin	No
Proerythroblast	15-20	Deep blue, opaque; no granules	Round, central; occupies about three-fourths of cell; deeply stained, uniformly granular texture	Yes
Basophilic erythroblast	12-16	Deep blue, opaque; may have blotchy appearance; no granules	Round, central occupies about half of cell; coarsely clumped, deeply stained	No
Polychromatophilic erythroblast	10-12	Variable, blue gray to slate gray	Round, dense, compact, deeply stained	No
Acidophilic erythroblast	8-10	Pink or pink with slight blue-gray	Round, dense, pyknotic, often eccentric	No
Lymphocyte	4-8	Thin rim of transparent blue cytoplasm	Deeply stained, round, slightly indented on one side	Yes
Monocyte	12-20	Opaque bluish gray with azurophilic granules	Large, kidney or horseshoe shaped	Yes
Plasma cell	6-20	Deeply basophilic except for prominent negative Golgi image	Eccentrically placed round to oval nucleus; coarse heterochromatin blocks	Yes

Heart

The wall of the heart consists of an inner lining layer (endocardium), a thick middle muscular layer (myocardium), and an external layer (epicardium).

Learning objectives for the heart:

1. Be able to recognize and describe the endocardium, myocardium and epicardium as well cardiac muscle cells and Purkinje fibers.

Endocardium

Examine a section from the interior of a heart chamber. The endocardium consists of a single layer of **endothelial cells** with oval or round nuclei that rests on a continuous layer of fine collagen fibers, separated from it by a thin basement membrane. This fibrous layer is the **subendothelial layer**. Just beneath it is a thicker layer of denser connective tissue that forms the majority of endocardium, the **subendocardial layer**. In addition to collagen fibers, it contains some elastic fibers, some smooth muscle cells, small blood vessels and, in the ventricles, may contain specialized cardiac muscle cells of the electrical conducting system. The connective tissue of the subendocardial layer binds the endocardium to the cardiac muscle of the myocardium.

Myocardium

The myocardium consists mainly of **cardiac muscle cells**. It is thickest in the left ventricle and thinnest in the atria. Note that the fine connective tissue enveloping each cardiac muscle cell of the ventricular myocardium contains numerous capillaries. In the atria, bundles of cardiac muscle are prominent adjacent to the lumen and form the **pectinate muscles**. Isolated bundles of cardiac muscle that project into the lumen of the ventricles form the **trabeculae carnea**. In the atria, cardiac muscle cells are smaller than elsewhere in the heart. Elastic fibers are scarce in the ventricular myocardium but are plentiful in the atria where they form an interlacing network between cardiac muscle cells. Here the elastic fibers of the myocardium become continuous with those of the endocardium and epicardium.

Epicardium

The epicardium is the **visceral layer** of the **pericardium**. The free surface is covered by a single layer of flat to cuboidal **mesothelial cells**, beneath which is a layer of connective tissue rich in elastic fibers. Adjacent to the myocardium, it contains blood vessels, nerves and an abundance of fat cells. This region is referred to as the **subepicardial layer**.

Make a labeled sketch demonstrating the entire ventricular wall and illustrate all three layers.

Cardiac skeleton

The cardiac skeleton consists of several connective tissue structures to which the cardiac musculature is attached. The most significant portion is formed by the **annuli fibrosi**, rings of dense connective tissue that surround the openings of the pulmonary artery and aorta. Masses of fibrous connective tissue, the **trigona fibrosi**, occur between the atrioventricular and atrial openings and the **septum membranaceum** (the upper fibrous part of the interventricular septum) also contribute to the cardiac skeleton. These structures consist of dense collagen fibers, scattered elastic fibers and occasional fat cells. With aging, portions of the cardiac skeleton may calcify.

Valves

Valves occur between the atria and ventricles and at the openings of the aorta and pulmonary vessels. All show a similar microscopic morphology. The **atrioventricular valves** are attached to annuli fibrosi, the connective tissue of which extends into each valve to form its core. The valves are covered on both sides by endocardium that is thicker on the ventricular side. Elastic fibers are prominent on the ventricular side of the valves whereas scattered smooth muscle cells are present in the endocardium on the atrial side. Thin tendinous cords called **chordae tendineae** attach the ventricular sides of the valves to projections of cardiac muscle called **papillary muscles**.

Make a sketch illustrating the relationship of the chordae tendineae to both a papillary muscle and an atrioventricular valve.

Conducting system

The conducting system of the heart consists of specialized cardiac muscle cells. Those of the atrioventricular bundle and its branches are called **Purkinje cells** (fibers). These specialized cardiac muscle cells are found in the subendocardial layer of the ventricles. Purkinje cells are larger and lighter staining than ordinary cardiac muscle cells and contain much more sarcoplasm.

Myofibrils are less abundant and usually have a peripheral location. Purkinje cells are rich in glycogen and mitochondria and often have two or more centrally positioned nuclei. Although intercalated discs are uncommon between cells, numerous desmosomes are scattered along cell boundaries. In contrast, **nodal cells** are smaller than ordinary cardiac muscle cells and contain fewer and poorly organized myofibrils. Intercalated discs are not observed between nodal cells.

Make a sketch emphasizing both the size and morphology, comparing Purkinje fibers with those of regular cardiac muscle cells found in the myocardium.

Blood vessels

As in the heart, the walls of blood vessels consist of three major tunics, or coats. From the lumen outward these are the tunica intima, tunica media and tunica adventitia.

Learning objectives for blood vessels:

1. Be able to recognize and describe the three coats (tunica intima, tunica media and tunica adventitia) and their subcomponents in the following classes of blood vessel: elastic (conducting) arteries, muscular (distributing) arteries, small arteries, arterioles, capillaries, venules, small veins, medium sized veins and large veins. Relate these structural differences to the classification of the vessel.

Elastic or conducting arteries

Included in this class are the aorta, common iliacs, pulmonary, brachiocephalic, subclavian and common carotid arteries. A major feature of this type of artery is the diameter of the lumen, which makes the wall of the vessel, appear thin. The **tunica intima** is relatively thick and lined by endothelium. The subendothelial layer is formed by loose connective tissue that contains elastic fibers and a few smooth muscle cells. The **tunica media** is the thickest layer and consists largely of 50 - 70 elastic laminae, each about 2 or 3 μm thick and spaced 5 - 20 μm apart. Elastic fibers connect successive laminae. Smooth muscle cells arranged circumferentially within a fine connective tissue occupy the spaces between laminae. The **tunica adventitia** is relatively thin and consists of bundles of collagen fibers and a few elastic fibers in a loose helical arrangement about the vessel. Because of their size, these vessels have their own vasculature (small arteries and veins), the **vasa vasorum**. The vasa vasorum form a plexus in the tunica adventitia and generally do not penetrate deeply into the media. Small nerve bundles also may be encountered in the tunica adventitia and these are referred to as nervi vascularis.

Muscular or distributing arteries

These form the largest class and, except for the elastic arteries, the named arteries fall into this category. Compared to the luminal diameter, the walls are thick. The thickness of the wall is due primarily to the large amount of smooth muscle in the tunica media.

The **tunica intima** is made up of an endothelium, a subendothelial layer and an internal elastic lamina. The **subendothelial layer** is similar to that of elastic arteries, but as the size of the vessel decreases this layer becomes thinner. It consists of fine collagen fibers, a few elastic fibers and scattered smooth muscle cells that are longitudinal in their orientation. The **internal elastic lamina** is a fenestrated band of elastin that forms a prominent, scalloped boundary between the tunica intima and tunica media. The **tunica media** forms the thickest coat and consists mainly of smooth muscle cells arranged in concentric, helical layers around the lumen of the vessel. The number of smooth muscle layers varies from 10 to 40 in muscular arteries. Elastic tissue forms a second prominent fenestrated membrane, the **external elastic lamina**, at the junction of the tunica media and tunica adventitia.

The **tunica adventitia** is prominent in muscular arteries and in some cases may be as thick as the media. It consists primarily of collagen and elastic fibers that exhibit a longitudinal orientation to the vessel wall.

Small arteries and arterioles

These vessels differ from muscular arteries only in size and the thickness of their walls. The distinction between arterioles and small arteries is primarily one of definition. The tunica media of small arteries consists of 10 or less layers of smooth muscle cells. **Arterioles** are those small arteries in which the media contains only one or two layers of smooth muscle cells. The diameter of the arteriole is less than 300 μm. A subendothelial layer is lacking and the **tunica intima** consists only of **endothelium** and a fenestrated **internal elastic lamina**. At a diameter of 30 μm, the **tunica media** of arterioles consists of a single layer of circumferentially oriented smooth muscle cells. The internal elastic lamina is thin and disappears in terminal arterioles; a definite external elastic lamina is absent. The **tunica adventitia** also decreases in thickness, becoming very thin in the smallest arterioles.

Make a labeled sketch illustrating a segment of vessel wall that compares the structure of conducting, distributing, small arteries and arterioles.

How are these vessels similar? How do they differ?

Capillaries

Capillaries are the smallest functional units of the blood vascular system and lie between the arterial and venous limbs of the circulation. Their lumina range from 5 to 10 μm in diameter and in the smallest may be surrounded by a single endothelial cell. In capillaries of larger caliber, three to four endothelial cells may encompass the lumen. The **tunica intima** consists of endothelium and a basement membrane; the **tunica media is absent** and the tunica adventitia is greatly reduced. The **tunica adventitia** contains some collagen and elastic fibers embedded in a small amount of ground substance. Mast cells, macrophages and fibroblasts may also be present in this layer.

Veins

Veins carry blood from capillary beds to the heart and in their progression gradually increase in size and their walls thicken. Three coats - tunica intima, tunica media and tunica adventitia - can be distinguished but these are not as clearly defined as in arteries. Veins vary in structure much more than arteries and the thickness of the wall does not always relate to its size. Their walls generally are thinner due to a reduction of muscular and elastic components. Because their walls are less sturdy, veins tend to collapse when empty and in histologic sections may appear flattened, with irregular, slit-like lumina. Although the histologic classification of veins is less satisfactory than for arteries, several subdivisions usually are made: venules and small, medium, and large veins.

Venules

Venules form from the union of several capillaries to form vessels 10 - 50 μm in diameter. The **tunica intima** consists of a thin, continuous endothelium that lies on a thin basement membrane. A **tunica media** is absent in the smallest venules and the **thin tunica adventitia** consists only of a few collagen fibers and scattered fibroblasts. Mast cells, macrophages and plasma cells also may be found. As venules reach a diameter of about 50 μm, circularly oriented, scattered smooth muscle cells begin to appear and form a discontinuous, incomplete tunica media. The tunica adventitia also increases in thickness and is formed primarily by longitudinally arranged collagen fibers that form an open spiral around the venule.

Small veins

Small veins range from about 0.2 to 1.0 mm in diameter. A continuous endothelium that lies on a thin basement membrane continues to from the **tunica intima**. The **tunica media** contains one to four layers of smooth muscle cells separated by a thin network of collagen and elastic fibers. **Tunica adventitia** is a relatively thick coat, made up of longitudinally oriented collagen and some thin elastic fibers.

Medium veins

Veins classified as medium veins include most of the named veins except those forming major trunks. They range in size from 1 to 10 mm in diameter. The **tunica intima** is thin and consists of endothelial cells and a supporting basement membrane. A narrow subendothelial layer may be present and consists of fine collagen fibers and scattered thin elastic fibers. The latter may form a network at the junction between intima and media, however, a poorly defined internal elastic lamina is formed only in the larger vessels. The **tunica media** of most medium sized veins, though well developed, is thinner than in corresponding arteries. It consists of longitudinally arranged smooth muscle cells and collagen fibers. The **tunica adventitia** forms the thickest layer of the vessel wall. It consists of collagen and elastic fibers and often contains longitudinally oriented smooth muscle cells. Vasa vasorum are a feature in the larger vessels of this class. Most medium veins are equipped with **valves**. These structures form from pocket-like-flaps of tunica intima that project into the lumen of the vessel with their free edges oriented in the direction of blood flow. Valves consist of a core of connective tissue covered on both sides by endothelium. The connective tissue beneath the endothelium on the down-stream side of the valves contains a rich network of elastic fibers.

Large veins

In large veins such as the venae cavae, renal, external iliac, splenic, portal and mesenteric veins, the **tunica adventitia** forms the larger part of the wall. The tunica adventitia consists of a loosely knit connective tissue with thick, longitudinal bundles of collagen and elastic fibers. Layers of smooth muscle cells are present and show a longitudinal orientation in the **tunica media** of the inferior vena cava. The tunica media often is poorly developed (and may even be absent) in many large veins and has the same organization as that in medium veins. **Tunica intima** is supported by a subendothelial layer, which may become prominent in the larger trunks.

Make a labeled sketch comparing the structure of the wall observed in venules and small, medium and large veins.

Lymph vascular system

The lymph vascular system begins in most tissues as blindly ending lymph capillaries that drain into larger collecting vessels. This system recovers intercellular fluid not picked up by the blood vascular system and returns it to the blood. The lymphatic capillaries drain into larger collecting vessels, which then form two major lymphatic trunks. Lymph nodes occur in the course of these vessels and filter the lymph. Lymphatics are absent in bone marrow, the central nervous system, coats of the eye, internal ear and placenta.

Lymph capillaries

Lymph capillaries begin as blind tubes that branch and anastomose freely to form an extensive network in tissues and organs. They are thin-walled, wider and more irregular in shape than blood capillaries. The wall of a lymph capillary consists only of a **thin continuous endothelium** and a discontinuous basement membrane. The endothelium is surrounded by a small amount of collagenous connective tissue.

Collecting lymph vessels

Collecting lymph vessels differ from lymph capillaries both in size and the thickness of their walls. Although an intima, media and adventitia are described they are not clearly delineated. **Tunica intima** is composed of an endothelium supported by a thin network of longitudinally arranged elastic fibers. **Tunica media** consists primarily of circularly arranged smooth muscle cells but some run longitudinally. A few fine elastic fibers lie between muscle cells. The thickest coat is the **tunica adventitia**, which is composed of bundles of collagen fibers, elastic fibers and a few smooth muscle cells. All have a longitudinal orientation in the vessel wall. **Valves** are numerous in lymphatic vessels and as in veins arise in pairs as folds of the intima.

Lymphatic trunks

Collecting lymphatic vessels combine to form two main lymphatic trunks: the thoracic duct and right lymphatic trunk. Their structure generally resembles that of a large vein. **Tunica intima** is formed by a continuous endothelium and a subendothelial layer of fibroelastic tissue containing smooth muscle cells. Near the media elastic fibers converge into a thin internal elastic lamina. The **tunica media** is the thickest layer and contains more smooth muscle cells than does the tunica media of large veins. The smooth muscle cells are predominately circular in arrangement and are separated by collagenous tissue that contains some elastic fibers. **Tunica adventitia** is poorly defined and consists of bundles of longitudinally arranged collagen and elastic fibers, and occasional smooth muscle cells. Vas vasorum occur in the wall of the thoracic duct.

An excellent place to look for smaller caliber blood vessels and lymphatic vessels is in the adventitia of the gall bladder.

Table 9. Key histologic features of arteries and veins.

Arteries	Tunica intima	Tunica media	Tunica adventitia	Other
Large (elastic, conducting)	Thick subendothelial layer with elastic fibers and smooth muscle cells; prominent internal elastic lamina	Major coat, 50-70 elastic laminae; smooth muscle cells in a fine connective tissue between laminae	Thin, no external elastic lamina	Vasa vasorum extend through adventitia and about one-third of the way through media
Medium (muscular, distributing)	Thin subendothelial layer; prominent internal elastic lamina	Major coat; up to 40 layers of smooth muscle, some elastic tissue	May equal thickness of media; external elastic lamina present	These are the muscular (distributing) arteries including most of the named arteries
Small	Same	10 layers or less in small	Same	
Arteriole	Thin, lacks defined subendothelial layer, internal elastic lamina present	Forms the main coat, 1-2 layers of smooth muscle	Thin, fibroelastic, no external elastic lamina	Wall (relative to lumen) is thicker than any other vessel
Capillaries				
Continuous	Endothelium, pericytes	Absent	Scant reticular fibers	Diameter 5-10 μm
Fenestrated	Fenestrated endothelium	Absent	Scant reticular fibers	Found in glomerular capillaries or in capillaries of endocrine glands
Sinusoids	Attenuated endothelium, may be separated by gaps, discontinuous basal lamina	Absent	Scant reticular fibers	Wide lumina, irregular in outline; found in spleen and bone marrow
Veins				
Venule	Endothelium only; no internal elastic lamina	Very thin, 1-2 layers of smooth muscle cells in larger venules	Thin, compared with total wall	Diameter 10-50 μm
Medium, small	Thin, subendothelial layer lacking in smaller veins	Thin layer of smooth muscle, elastic and collagen fibers	Well developed, thick fibroelastic layer; no external elastic lamina	Valves present; medium 1-10 mm in diameter; small 0.2-1.0 mm in diameter
Large	Thicker than in small veins; a delicate internal elastic lamina may be present	Thin or even lacking	Thickest coat, fibromuscular; no external elastic lamina	Vasa vasorum

CHAPTER 9. LYMPHATIC ORGANS

Lymphatic organs consist of accumulations of nodular and diffuse lymphatic tissue organized into discrete structures that are isolated from surrounding tissues by a well defined capsule. A key to understanding their structure is to know generally what function they perform.

Learning objectives for the lymphatic organs:

1. Be able identify and describe the histologic detail of a tonsil and distinguish between tonsils.
2. Be able to identify and describe the histologic architecture of a lymph node. Be able to trace both the flow of lymph and blood through a lymph node.
3. Be able to identify and describe the histologic architecture of the spleen. Be able to trace the blood flow through the structure of the spleen and relate this flow to spleen function.
4. Be able to identify and describe the histologic architecture of the thymus. Be able to relate the structure of this lymphatic organ to its function.

Tonsils

Tonsils are aggregates of lymphatic nodules associated with the oropharynx, nasopharynx and tongue and form the palatine, pharyngeal and lingual tonsils, respectively. Tonsils do not filter lymph but do contribute to the formation of lymphocytes.

    Palatine tonsils are paired, oval lymphoid organs located laterally at the junction of the oropharynx and oral cavity. A **stratified squamous epithelium** covers the free surface of this tonsil and is very closely associated with the lymphatic tissue. Deep invaginations of this epithelium form **tonsillar crypts** that extend almost to the base of the tonsil. **Lymphatic nodules,** many with prominent **germinal centers**, are usually arranged in a single layer beneath the epithelium. The nodules are embedded in a mass of **diffuse lymphatic tissue**. A **partial capsule** of collagenous fibers beneath the basal surface of the tonsil separates it from surrounding structures. **Septa** of loosely arranged collagen fibers extend from the capsule into the tonsillar tissue and partially divide the tonsillar crypts and their associated lymphatic tissue from one another. Reticular fibers form the supporting framework (stroma) for the lymphatic tissue. Small mucous glands may be found, on occasion, lying just beyond the limiting capsule.

    Lingual tonsils lie in the root of the tongue and are similar in general structure to the palatine tonsils. Crypts that invaginate from the free surface are deep, may be branched and are lined by **stratified squamous epithelium**. Nodular and diffuse lymphatic tissues are closely associated with the epithelium. Mucous glands (posterior lingual minor salivary glands) embedded in **skeletal muscle** may be encountered just beyond a partial capsule of collagenous connective tissue.

    Pharyngeal tonsils are located on the posterior wall of the nasopharynx. The free (luminal) surface is covered by **ciliated pseudostratified columnar epithelium** that contains goblet cells. The crypts are not as deep as those associated with the palatine tonsils. **Note:** Patches of stratified squamous epithelium may be present in the surface-covering epithelium and tend to become a more common observation with aging, in smokers and in those subject to chronic infection. By viewing the epithelium lining the crypts, the identity of the surface-lining epithelium can be checked. If ciliated pseudostratified columnar epithelium is encountered, then the tonsil in question must be pharyngeal in origin. A **thin capsule** of collagen fibers separates the nodular and diffuse lymphatic tissue from underlying structures.

Make a labeled sketch comparing the palatine and pharyngeal tonsils.

Lymph nodes

Lymph nodes are small encapsulated lymphatic organs set in the course of lymphatic vessels to **filter lymph**. They usually are flattened, bean-shaped structures with a slight indentation on one side called the **hilum**. To best understand the structure of a lymph node examine the supporting framework first. The surrounding thin **capsule** consists of closely packed collagen fibers and scattered elastic fibers. A few smooth muscle cells can be found at the entrance and exit points of lymphatic vessels. Thin **trabeculae** of dense irregular connective tissue extend from the inner surface of the capsule into the interior of the lymph node. The areas enclosed by the capsule and trabeculae are filled by a network of **reticular fibers** and their associated **reticular cells**. The latter are modified fibroblasts that produce and maintain reticular fibers. The reticular fiber network can be seen only following special (silver) staining techniques. Using the low power objective observe the **arrangement** of the **diffuse** and **nodular lymphatic tissue**. The **cortex** forms a layer beneath the capsule that extends for a variable distance toward the interior of the lymph node. It consists of **lymphatic nodules,** several with germinal centers, set in a bed of **diffuse lymphatic tissue**. Trabeculae run perpendicular to the capsule and separate the cortex into several incomplete compartments.

The cortex can also be subdivided according to the type of lymphatic tissue it contains. The **outer cortex** contains nodular and diffuse lymphatic tissue. The **deep (inner) cortex** consists only of diffuse lymphatic tissue. There is no sharp boundary between these two zones and their proportions differ from node to node and with the functional status of a given node. An appreciation of these two zones is important because B-lymphocytes tend to be concentrated in the outer nodular lymphatic tissue, while T lymphocytes are present in the diffuse lymphatic tissue of the deep cortex. The deep cortex is depleted of cells after thymectomy and for this reason is often referred to as the thymus-dependent area. **Follicular dendritic cells** are found in this area and can be identified by their pale-staining nuclei and numerous long cytoplasmic processes. The deep cortex continues into the medulla without a clear boundary or interruption. At low power the **medulla** appears as a pale staining area of variable width that surrounds a region of the node with a slight indentation called the hilus. The medulla consists of **diffuse lymphatic tissue** arranged as irregular branching **medullary cords**. The medullary cords contain abundant lymphocytes, macrophages and plasma cells. With high power, study and examine several macrophages containing phagocytosed material and review the cytologic features of plasma cells. Return to the low-power objective and note that the trabeculae in the medulla are more irregularly arranged than those of the cortex.

Now scan the lymph node for **lymph sinuses**. It must be kept in mind that the lymph node is designed to filter lymph. The lymph sinuses are a system of channel-like spaces through which lymph percolates. Lymph enters the node through afferent lymphatic vessels that can pierce the capsule anywhere along the concave border and empty into a narrow space that separates the capsule and cortex, the **subcapsular (marginal) sinus**. Examine the external surface of the capsule for afferent lymphatic vessels. These dilated, endothelial lined vessels have **valves** that project into the lumen. The valves of **afferent** vessels open **toward** the node; those of **efferent** vessels open **away from** the node. Move to the hilus and also find and examine efferent lymphatic vessels and any valves present. Return to the subcapsular sinus and note while examining this space with the high-power objective that it does not form a tubular structure but is a wide space extending beneath the capsule. The subcapsular sinus is **continuous** with the **trabecular (cortical, intermediate) sinuses** that lie adjacent to trabeculae and extend radially into the cortex. Trabecular sinuses are in turn continuous with **medullary sinuses** that run between the medullary cords of the medulla. At the hilus, the subcapsular and medullary sinuses pierce the capsule and become continuous with efferent lymphatic vessels. The three sinuses are continuous one with the other and show similar morphologic features. Examine stellate cells (reticular cells) supported by fine reticular fibers that criss-cross the lumen of the sinuses and are joined to each other by slender processes. Numerous macrophages are present in this luminal network and extend from boundaries of the sinuses. The flattened cells that form the margins of the sinuses are regarded as attenuated endothelial cells, akin to those that line lymphatic vessels with which they are continuous. Observe that the sinuses in the cortex are narrower and less numerous than those in the medulla. Sinuses in the medulla are large, irregular and repeated branch and anastomose separating medullary cords. Return to low power and trace the blood supply of the lymph node, which enters and exits the node through the hilus. **Arteries** (arterioles) from the hilus at first lie within medullary trabeculae but soon leave these structures and enter the medullary cords as they course toward the cortex. In the cortex they break up into a capillary plexus that supplies the diffuse and nodular lymphatic tissue. The capillaries then join to form venules that run from the cortex to enter medullary cords as **small veins**. These in turn combine to form larger veins that leave at the hilus. Return to and **examine the deep cortex**. Here, venules have a special appearance and are called **post-capillary venules**. Post-capillary venules are characterized by a high endothelium that varies from cuboidal to columnar in shape, often occluding the lumen. Small lymphocytes are often seen passing through the walls of these vessels. Post-capillary venules can be found by looking for light-staining minute duct-like structures superimposed against the blue background of lymphocyte nuclei.

Make a detailed sketch of an entire lymph node and label its subcomponents.

Spleen

Unlike lymph nodes, the primary function of the spleen is to **filter blood**. Therefore, the **spleen lacks** afferent lymphatics and lymphatic sinuses and **is not** arranged into a cortex and medulla. Because it filters blood, the spleen has a distinctive pattern of blood circulation and specialized channels that facilitate blood filtration. The lymphatic tissue associated with the spleen is arranged about this vascular pattern. Prior to putting a preparation of spleen under the microscope examine it visually and observe that it is solid mass of tissue, one that has been cut out of a much larger structure. Note too, the scattered regions of basophilic material visible within the section.

Framework of spleen

The spleen is limited by a **well-developed capsule** of dense irregular connective tissue. Elastic fibers are present and most abundant in the deeper layers and groups of smooth muscle cells may be encountered but their number is variable. Broad bands of connective tissue, the **trabeculae**, extend from the inner surface of the capsule and form a rich, branching anastomosing framework in the interior of the spleen. The region between trabeculae is filled by a network of reticular fibers and cells. Appreciate that this supporting reticular network cannot be seen in H&E preparations but can be demonstrated by special silver impregnation techniques. In routine preparations, at low power, note that the substance of the spleen (splenic pulp) lying between trabeculae consists of differentially stained regions that also are of different morphology. Identify the scattered regions of nodular lymphatic tissue, which stains more deeply basophilic due to the greater concentration of lymphocyte nuclei. This is the **white pulp**. The white pulp is surrounded by **diffuse lymphatic tissue suffused with blood** that imparts a reddish color to this region due to the large number of erythrocytes present. This area of the splenic pulp is called the **red pulp**.

Blood supply of the spleen

The internal architecture of the spleen is best explained by first understanding its relationship to the blood circulation. The nodular lymphatic tissue of the **white pulp** generally is associated with the **arterial supply** of the spleen. The diffuse lymphatic tissue of the **red pulp** is associated with the **venous system** of the spleen.

Branches of the splenic artery enter the spleen at the hilus, divide and travel within trabeculae into the interior of the spleen. The small arteries within trabeculae are called **trabecular arteries**. Locate a trabecula and a contained trabecular artery and examine each carefully. Branches of the trabecular artery eventually leave the trabecula as **central arteries** and as they do immediately become surrounded by a sleeve of lymphatic tissue termed the **periarterial lymphatic sheath (PALS)**. Where the sheath expands to form **lymphatic nodules** the **central** (follicular arteriole) **artery** is usually displaced to one side (despite its name) and assumes an eccentric position within the nodule. The lymphatic nodules may or may not show a central, lighter staining **germinal center**. The lymphatic nodules of the spleen also are known as **splenic follicles** or Malphigian corpuscles. The periarterial lymphatic sheaths and the splenic follicles make up the **white pulp** of the spleen. Throughout its course in the white pulp, the central artery provides numerous capillaries to the surrounding lymphatic tissue, which then pass into a **marginal zone** surrounding the white pulp. How the capillaries end is unknown. Examine the marginal zone carefully. It lies at the boundary of the white pulp and consists of a thin zone of reticular fibers and cells more closely meshed than elsewhere into thin concentric layers that limit the lymphatic tissue of the white pulp from the red pulp. Interdigitating (dendritic-like) cells are present in this region. Attempt to trace the stem of the central artery as it leaves the white pulp and passes into a splenic cord of the **red pulp**. Here it divides into several short, straight **penicillar arteries**. Some of these will acquire a surrounding layer of concentrically arranged cells and fibers and are called **sheathed capillaries**. Cells within the sheath are avidly phagocytic. Not all capillaries are sheathed and occasionally one sheath may enclose more than one capillary.

The next element of the splenic circulation to be identified should be the splenic sinusoids. **Splenic sinusoids** separate the diffuse lymphatic tissue of the red pulp into a network of branching, cord-like structures called **splenic cords**. The sinusoids have wide lumina (20 - 40 μm in diameter) and their walls are unique, being made up of elongated, fusiform **endothelial cells** oriented parallel to the long axis of the sinusoid. The endothelial cells lie side by side around the sinusoidal lumen but are not in contact and are separated by **small spaces**. These cells are supported only by **bars of basement membrane** (rather than a continuous sheath) that spiral around and encircle the sinusoid to aid in holding the endothelial cells in three-dimensional space. With special staining (periodic acid-Schiff) these bars of basement membrane can be demonstrated. Examine the walls of several splenic sinusoids carefully with the high-power objective. In some preparations, particularly when the sinusoids are filled with blood, the walls of the sinusoids may be difficult to observe. If this is the case, using the high-power objective examine the red pulp for the following: look for a chain (five to seven in a row) of light-staining nuclei each separated from its neighbor by a small space. These are transverse sections through endothelial cell nuclei comprising a sinusoidal wall. The wall of a splenic sinusoid can be traced by looking for these chains of nuclei. At times, a thin, hair-like strand of material can be seen on the external surface of the sinusoids. These strands are the bars of basement membrane. Examine a scanning electron micrograph illustrating the three-dimensional configuration of a splenic sinusoid to affirm a mental image of this structure. Re-examine the splenic cords of the red pulp. Note the large number of erythrocytes present, which imparts the color of the red pulp.

The meshwork of reticular fibers and cells is continuous throughout the red pulp and is filled with a large number of free cells including all those found in blood. Confirm the presence of erythrocytes, lymphocytes, granular leukocytes and platelets within the splenic cords. **Macrophages** also can be observed that contain ingested erythrocytes or may be laden with a yellowish brown pigment, **hemosiderin**, formed from the breakdown of hemoglobin.

Make a detailed sketch of the spleen and label the various subcomponents observed.

Thymus

The thymus is the only lobulated lymphatic organ. The thymus functions **not** in the filtering of lymph or blood **but in** the **production of lymphocytes**, the T lymphocytes. Morphologically, the thymus consists of two lobes joined by connective tissue. A **thin capsule** of loosely woven collagen fibers envelopes each lobe and gives rise to **fine septa** that extend into the thymus, subdividing each lobe into a number of irregular shaped **lobules**. With low power, note that each lobule consists of an outer, darker-staining **cortex** surrounding a central, light staining **medulla**. The medullary region of each lobule is continuous with that of adjacent lobules throughout the thymus. Does your section confirm this continuity? The free cells (primarily lymphocytes) are contained within a reticular network (stroma) as in the lymph node and spleen, however, that of the **thymus differs markedly** from the other lymphatic organs. The stroma of the thymus consists of a **cytoreticulum** composed of epithelial cells rather than reticular fibers. These **epithelial reticular cells** are stellate in shape with long, thin cytoplasmic processes that are linked to processes of other reticular cells and are at their points of contact united by **desmosomes**. Thus, the free cells are supported by the cytoplasmic processes of the reticular cells and **not by** reticular fibers. Although these processes are obscured by lymphocytes and other cells, the epithelial reticular cells can be identified by their large, round or oval euchromatic nuclei that may contain one or more prominent nucleoli. The surrounding cytoplasm is light staining and irregular in shape. Reticular fibers in the thymus are found only in relation to blood vessels.

Carefully examine a central region of the cortex with the high-power objective. Note that most cells of the cortex are small lymphocytes. The dark basophilia of this region is the result of the high concentration of lymphocyte nuclei. Examine the region of the outer cortex immediately interior to the capsule for large, medium and small lymphocytes as well as mitotic figures. **Large lymphocytes** tend to concentrate in the outer cortex immediately beneath the capsule where they can be found in small numbers. They are large, round or oval shaped cells with large euchromatic nuclei and prominent nucleoli. As with **medium-sized lymphocytes** in this region, they both exhibit lymphoid characteristics (overall shape and character of nucleus) but differ in size, shape and lighter staining of the nucleus. Medium-sized lymphocytes are about twice the size of adjacent small lymphocytes and exhibit a considerable amount of light-staining cytoplasm. Large lymphocytes may be four times the size of small lymphocytes. The nuclei also are lighter staining as compared to small lymphocytes. Scattered among the small lymphocytes slightly deeper in the cortex, look for cells in mitosis as considerable mitotic activity occurs in this region and several **mitotic figures** should be found.

The **medulla** forms the pale central region of the thymus. Lymphocytes are less numerous than in the cortex. Epithelial reticular cells tend to be pleomorphic and are numerous. The majority of free cells in the medulla are small lymphocytes but small, variable numbers of macrophages, mast cells and eosinophilic granulocytes can also be found. Find and compare these various cell types. The most prominent feature in the medulla is the **thymic (Hassall's) corpuscles**. These bodies vary from 10 to 100 μm or more in diameter and consist of flattened epithelial reticular cells, wrapped around one another in concentric lamellations. Many contain keratohyalin granules. Cells at the center of some corpuscles undergo hyalinization or necrosis. Confirm previous identifications of epithelial reticular cells of the stroma by comparing these healthy cells (particularly the nuclei) with those constituting the corpuscles.

Make a detailed, labeled sketch of the thymus, including the position of large and medium-sized lymphocytes as well as mitotic figures.

Table 10. Key histologic features of lymphatic organs.

	Tonsil	Lymph node	Spleen	Thymus
Capsule	Partial, at base	Yes	Yes	Thin
Trabeculae	No	Yes	Yes	Forms thin septa
Lymphatic tissue arranged as cortex and medulla	No	Yes	No	Yes
Nodular lymphatic tissue	Yes	Yes	Yes	No
Special features	Crypts; closely associated with overlying epithelium **Palatine** and **Lingual**: non keratinized stratified squamous **Pharyngeal**: ciliated pseudostratified columnar	Subcapsular, trabecular and medullary sinuses; only lymphatic organ with afferent and efferent lymphatics	Lymphatic tissue arranged as red and white pulp; splenic follicles (nodules) associated with central arteries; sinusoids in red pulp	Thymic corpuscles in medulla; stroma is a cytoreticulum of endodermal origin

The skin consists of an epithelium (keratinized stratified squamous) called the epidermis and an underlying layer of connective tissue called the dermis. The appendages of skin (hair, nails, sweat and sebaceous glands) together with the two components of skin form the **integument**. The terms **thick** and **thin skin** refer to the thickness of the epidermis and not to the thickness of the skin as a whole.

Learning objectives for the integument:

1. Be able to identify the strata comprising the epidermis of both thick and thin skin. Recognize the morphological changes that occur in the keratinocyte as it passes through the various strata of the epidermis. Identify three other cell types that also occur in the epidermis.
2. Be able to identify the two basic layers of the dermis and any associated subcomponents.
3. Be able to identify the appendages of skin and their structural subcomponents.

Epidermis

The epidermis consists of several layers (strata) that reflect a sequential differentiation of the **keratinocytes**, the primary epithelial cell type forming the epidermis. In thick skin, the layers are stratum basale, stratum spinosum, stratum granulosum, stratum lucidum and stratum corneum. In thin skin the layers are narrower and less well defined and the stratum lucidum absent.

The **stratum basale**, together with its basement membrane, abuts the underlying dermis and consists of a single row of columnar epithelial cells that follows the contours of the ridges and papillae. Note any mitotic figures that may be present. The adjacent overlying layer, **stratum spinosum**, consists of polyhedral cells that become somewhat flattened in the outermost layers. Cells of this layer are held tightly together by numerous desmosomes. During tissue preparation cells of this layer tend to shrink and pull apart slightly except at these points of attachment. As a result, the cells have numerous, short spiny projections that extend between adjacent cells. Because of their appearance, cells of this layer are often referred to as spiny or prickle cells. In thick skin the **stratum granulosum** consists of three to five layers of flattened cells whose long axes lie parallel to the surface. Cells of this layer are characterized by numerous dark staining **keratohyalin granules**. At the surface of stratum granulosum lies a narrow, undulating lightly stained zone known as the **stratum lucidum**. This narrow layer consists of several layers

of cells so compacted together that outlines of individual cells cannot be distinguished. Impressions of flattened nuclei may be seen, but usually this layer is characterized by a lack of nuclei. **Stratum corneum** forms the outermost layer of the epidermis and consists of scalelike cells called **squames**. Squames represent the remains of cells that have lost their nuclei, all organelles and desmosomal attachments to adjacent cells. They are filled with **keratin**. The outermost squames of stratum corneum are constantly shed and this region often is referred to as the **stratum disjunctum.**

Three other cell types are associated with the epidermis but are fewer in number. **Melanocytes** are scattered throughout the basal layer and send processes that extend between the cells of stratum spinosum. Melanocytes produce **melanin granules** (melanosomes), a brown pigment that imparts shades of brown to black color to the skin. Melanocytes transfer melanosomes to the cytoplasm of adjacent keratinocytes, which exhibit melanin granules when viewed under the microscope. The melanocytes producing this pigment may actually contain less melanin than neighboring keratinocytes and appear light in color. **Langerhans s cells**, although present throughout the epidermis, are most frequently encountered in the upper region of the stratum spinosum. In H&E sections they have darkly stained, large convoluted nuclei surrounded by a clear cytoplasm. Using special stains Langerhans cells appear as stellate (dendritic) cells and present a morphology typical of antigen-presenting cells. **Merkel s cells** are the least numerous and tend to lie close to nerve endings in the stratum basale and are distinguished by indented nuclei and a light staining cytoplasm with dust-like granules.

Dermis

The dermis is arranged into superficial papillary and deep reticular layers. The **papillary layer** lies immediately beneath the epidermis. It is a thin layer and continues into the **dermal papillae**. These are small conical projections of fine connective tissue that extend between **epidermal ridges**. The latter are complementary projections of the epidermis into the underlying dermis. Collagen fibers and bundles tend to be thin and loosely arranged in the papillary layer. In contrast, the **reticular layer** is the thicker, denser part of the dermis. It consists of larger interwoven bundles of collagen, closely packed together and is typical dense irregular connective tissue. The two layers are not clearly demarcated from one another. Identify the numerous capillary loops present in the connective tissue of the dermal papillae. In some, especially those in the palms and fingers, nerve endings and tactile corpuscles also are present. Find and examine a **Meissner s corpuscle**.

This tactile corpuscle is characterized by a supporting framework that whorls about a centrally positioned nerve ending. Examine the deeper regions of the reticular layer and adjacent hypodermis for any **Pacinian corpuscles** that may be present.

Make a labeled sketch comparing sections of thick and thin skin.

Appendages of the skin

Appendages of the skin include nails, hair, sebaceous and sweat glands. All are derived from the epidermis.

Nail

Nails are hard, keratinized structures that cover the dorsal surfaces of the tips of the fingers and toes. The **nail** consists of a visible **nail plate** (body) and a **root** implanted in a groove in the skin. The nail plate is a modification of the cornified zone of the epidermis and consists of several layers of flattened cells with degenerate nuclei. The cells are tightly adherent, clear and translucent. Beneath the nail plate lies the **nail bed**, which corresponds to the stratum spinosum and stratum basale of the epidermis. The underlying dermis is organized into numerous longitudinal vascular ridges. Near the root the ridges are smaller and less vascular. The pink color of nails is due to transmission of color from this underlying capillary bed. Near the root, the nail is more opaque and forms a crescentic area, the lunule. The nail bed beneath the root and lunule is thicker, actively proliferative and is concerned with the growth of the nail. This region is called the **nail matrix**. Note that cells in the deepest layer of the nail matrix are cylindrical in shape and show frequent mitoses.

Hair

Each hair consists of a root embedded in the skin and a hair shaft projecting above the surface of the epidermis. The **medulla** (core) of a hair shaft consists of flattened, cornified polyhedral cells in which the nuclei are pyknotic or missing. The bulk of the hair shaft consists of the **cortex**, formed by several layers of intensely cornified, elongated cells tightly compacted together. Pigment of colored hair is found in the cells and in intercellular spaces of the cortex. The outermost layer is thin and forms the **cuticle**. The cuticle consists of a single layer of clear, flattened squamous cells. With high power, observe that these cells overlap each other, shingle fashion, from below upwards.

The **root** expands to form the **hair bulb**, which is indented at its deep surface by a conical projection of vascular connective tissue called a **papilla**. Examine the lower part of the hair root and note that the cells of the cortex and medulla tend to be cuboidal in shape and contain nuclei of normal appearance. At upper levels in the root, nuclei become indistinct and are lost. Cells of the cortex become progressively flattened as they move toward the skin surface.

Hair follicle

Each hair root is enclosed within a tubular sheath called a hair follicle, which consists of an inner epithelial component and an outer connective tissue component. The epithelial component is derived from the epidermis and consists of inner and outer root sheaths. The connective tissue component is derived from the dermis.

The **inner epithelial root sheath** corresponds to the superficial layers of the epidermis that have undergone specialization to form three layers. The innermost layer is called the **cuticle of the root sheath**. The cells are thin and scalelike and are overlapped from above downward; the free edges of these cells interlock with the free edges of the cells forming the hair cuticle. Immediately adjacent to the cuticle of the root sheath are several layers of elongated cells that form **Huxley s layer**. These cells contain large **trichohyalin granules** that are reddish in appearance. A single row of clear, flattened cells surround Huxley s layer and is called **Henle s layer**. Cells comprising all three layers are nucleated in the distal parts, but as the sheath nears the surface, the nuclei are lost.

The **outer epithelial root sheath** is a direct continuation of stratum spinosum and stratum basale and show similar histological features. Examine a narrow clear zone, the **glassy membrane**, which lies between columnar epithelial cells forming the external surface of the outer epithelial root sheath and the surrounding **connective tissue sheath**. It is equivalent to the basement membrane of the epidermis.

Sebaceous glands

Generally, sebaceous glands are associated with hairs and drain into the upper part of hair follicles. In some regions they open directly onto the surface of the skin. Sebaceous glands vary in size and consist of a cluster of two to five oval alveoli drained by a single duct. The secretory alveoli lie within the dermis and are limited by a well-defined basement membrane. Cells abutting the basement membrane are small, cuboidal and contain round nuclei. Mitotic figures can be found among cells of this layer. **The entire alveolus is filled with cells**. Centrally, they become much larger, lighter staining and gradually accumulate lipid droplets in their cytoplasm. Near the duct, the nuclei of these large cells become pyknotic, degenerate and ultimately disappear. In this region the entire cell breaks down and the cell debris together with the lipid droplets form the secretory product called **sebum**. This type of secretion, in which the entire cell is the secretory product, is known as **holocrine secretion**. Note that the short duct of the sebaceous gland is lined by stratified squamous epithelium and drains into the lumen of an adjacent hair follicle. Sebaceous glands are closely associated with bundles of smooth muscle, the **arrector pili muscles**. Collectively, the hair follicle, hair shaft, sebaceous gland and arrector pili muscle is referred to as the **pilosebaceous apparatus**.

Sweat glands

Two classes of sweat glands occur: eccrine sweat glands, found in most regions of skin, and apocrine sweat glands, restricted primarily to the axilla, groin and circumanal region.

Eccrine sweat glands

These are generally distributed throughout most regions of skin in variable numbers. They are plentiful in the palms and soles and least numerous in the skin of the back and neck. Each is a simple coiled tubule, the deep region of which is tightly coiled and forms the secretory portion. It is often located deep within the dermis. The secretory unit consists of a simple columnar epithelium. Some cells forming this segment of the gland may exhibit a narrow apex and a broad base, others a broad apex and a narrow base. The duct is formed by stratified cuboidal epithelium that stains more deeply basophilic than the secretory portion. In the epidermis the duct consists of a spiral channel that is simply a cleft between epidermal cells; cells immediately adjacent to the lumen of the duct are circularly arranged. **Myoepithelial cells** are present around the secretory portion, situated between the basement membrane and the bases of the secretory cells. These stellate cells have nuclei similar in appearance to those of fibroblasts and light-staining processes. Myoepithelial cells are most easily seen in grazing sections of the secretory units. **Apocrine sweat glands** are enlarged, modified eccrine sweat glands. The tubular units are much larger, with very large open lumina. Associated myoepithelial cells also are larger and more numerous than those of eccrine sweat glands. The ducts are similar to those of ordinary sweat glands but empty into hair follicles rather than onto the surface of the epidermis.

Make a labeled sketch comparing eccrine and apocrine sweat glands to sebaceous glands.

How can each gland be classified?

	Epidermis	Dermis	Other
Thick skin	Shows five layers: stratum corneum very thick, stratum lucidum is present, stratum granulosum is 4-5 cells thick, and stratum spinosum and basale are prominent	Papillary and reticular layer well defined	Only on palms of hands, soles of feet; contains eccrine sweat glands, the only glands present in thick skin
Thin skin	Lacks a stratum lucidum; thin stratum corneum, stratum granulosum usually is a single layer of cells, and stratum spinosum is much thinner	As for thick skin, depth varies with area; thick dermis in skin between scapulae; delicate dermis over eyelids, scrotum, penis; thinner on anterior surface of body than on posterior surface	Contains hair follicles, sebaceous glands, and eccrine sweat glands; apocrine sweat glands in axilla and groin

Table 11. Key histologic features that distinguish thick and thin skin.

CHAPTER 11. DIGESTIVE SYSTEM

The digestive system consists of a large irregularly shaped tube, which is subdivided into the oral cavity, esophagus, stomach, small and large intestines, rectum and anal canal. Glands associated with this system that lie outside the digestive tube proper are connected to it by ducts. A good method for examining the digestive tube is to use a consistent method of examination and realize that this tube, except for the oral cavity, consists of four basic layers. Identification of each of these layers with the low-power objective, beginning at the luminal surface, is an important exercise in developing an understanding of this morphologically complex tube. The luminal-most layer is called the mucosa (mucous membrane) followed by an underlying submucosa of coarse connective tissue, a muscle wall and an outer layer of connective tissue that may or may not be associated with a simple squamous epithelium (mesothelium).

Learning objectives for the digestive system:

1. Be able to distinguish the different subdivisions of the digestive system.
2. Be able to recognize taste buds, the types of papillae, minor salivary glands and musculature associated with the tongue.
3. Be able to differentiate between the three major salivary glands according to their structure.
4. Be able to distinguish the subcomponents of adult and developing teeth and their associated cell types.
5. Be able to distinguish the four strata in each region of the tubular portion of the digestive system (alimentary canal). Recognize both the similarities and the differences of each region.
6. Be able to distinguish the primary junctions between regions (organs) that occur along the alimentary canal.

Oral cavity

The walls of the irregularly shaped oral cavity consist of the lips, cheeks, tongue, teeth, gingiva and palate. The mucosa lining the oral cavity is formed by a non-keratinized stratified squamous epithelium supported by a fine connective tissue layer called the lamina propria.

Lip

Examine a section of lip with the low-power objective and determine that it consists of a series of layers or strata. The mucosal (inner) surface can be identified by the thick lining of **nonkeratinized stratified squamous epithelium** overlying a **compact lamina propria**. Mixed mucoserous labial glands (a minor salivary gland) lie among the coarse connective tissue fibers of the next layer, the **submucosa**. The latter unites the mucosa to **skeletal muscle fibers** of the orbicularis oris muscle, which forms the center of the lip. Connective tissue fibers from the dermis unite typical thin skin to the external aspect of this muscle. Next, trace the covering thin skin (keratinized stratified squamous epithelium with associated sweat glands, hair follicles and sebaceous glands) to the vermilion border. Here the lip is covered by a non-keratinized stratified squamous epithelium that lacks hair follicles and glands. Note the numerous tall, vascular connective tissue papillae that project into the overlying epithelium providing this translucent region in life with a red hue. Note also that the epithelium lining the mucosal surface is considerably thicker than that of the epidermis.

Sketch the layers of the lip, as well as their sub-components, beginning with the mucosal surface.

Cheek and palate

Compare a section of cheek to that of the lip and observe that both exhibit similar histologic features. Identify and examine the subcomponents of the mucosa, submucosa, skeletal muscle (buccinator muscle) and typical thin skin. The submucosa of the cheek also contains mixed, minor salivary glands called buccal glands. In examining a section of soft palate proceed from the nonkeratinized stratified squamous epithelium and lamina propria facing the oral cavity to a submucosa, through skeletal muscle (palatine muscles) to a lamina propria supporting ciliated pseudostratified columnar epithelium with goblet cells lining the nasopharynx.

Tongue

Examine a section of tongue with the low-power objective and observe that the mucous membrane is firmly bound to a core of interwoven fascicles of skeletal muscle that run in three different planes, each perpendicular to the other. A submucosa is absent. Four types of papillae are associated with dorsal surface of the tongue. Identify the type of papillae present in the section of tongue being examined. **Filiform papillae** are thin papillae 2 - 3 mm long that contain a conical core of connective tissue continuous with that of the underlying lamina propria. The covering stratified squamous epithelium may show variable degrees of cornification. Filiform papillae are the most numerous of the papillae.

Fungiform papillae occur singly scattered between the filiform type. They are larger, dome-shaped and contain a connective tissue core rich in capillaries. In life, fungiform papillae appear as red dots on the dorsal surface of the tongue. They may or may not be associated with taste buds. The largest of the papillae, **circumvallate papillae**, are restricted in distribution to the V-shaped sulcus terminalis that divides the tongue into anterior and posterior regions. They number between 10 and 14 in man. Circumvallate papillae appear sunk into the mucosa of the tongue separated from a surrounding wall of lingual tissue by a deep furrow. **Serous** minor salivary glands within the tongue called **von Ebner s glands** lie in the lamina propria or between muscle fascicles and drain into the base of this furrow. A large core of connective tissue with numerous vessels, unmyelinated nerves and small serous glands fills the core of the circumvallate papillae. Observe that the epithelium covering the lateral surfaces of these papillae contains numerous taste buds. **Taste buds** appear as lightly stained, oval structures that extend from the surface of the lining epithelium to the basement membrane. Component cells are arranged like segments of an orange around a small **taste pore** that opens into the external environment at the epithelial surface. The component cells have large microvilli (taste hairs) that project into the taste pore. **Foliate papillae** are poorly developed in man but in some species (rabbits) appear as parallel ridges and furrows in the mucosa on the dorsolateral aspect of the tongue. Numerous taste buds occur in the epithelium lining the lateral surfaces of these papillae and serous glands empty into the bottoms of the adjacent furrows.

Sketch a taste bud within the lining epithelium of one of these papillae.

Major salivary glands

Compare and contrast the three major salivary glands: the parotid, submandibular and sublingual glands. **All are compound tubular alveolar glands**, as are all of the minor salivary glands associated with the oral cavity. Differences in histologic structure are due, primarily, to differences in the **proportion of cells (serous or mucous)** making up the secretory units **and lengths** of various segments of the **intralobular duct system**.

The secretory units of the **parotid gland** are made up **entirely of serous** secretory cells. The parotid is enclosed in a fibrous capsule and is subdivided into lobes and lobules by connective tissue septa extending from the capsule. Note the abundant, scattered fat cells in the connective tissue between the secretory units. Scan the section carefully and sketch

the fine connective tissue septa that circumscribe individual lobules. Examine the interior of the lobule and confirm that the secretory tubules and alveoli are composed of pyramidal serous cells with basally placed, oval nuclei, basophilic cytoplasm and discrete apical secretory granules. Identify **intercalated ducts**, the initial segment of the duct system, lined by a simple squamous or low cuboidal epithelium. These are tiny ducts and may show only four or five cells organized around a minute lumen. They exhibit a staining intensity similar to the secretory units. Identify **striated ducts**, which are lined by cuboidal or columnar cells that exhibit numerous **basal striations**. These are considerably larger than the intercalated ducts and the simple cuboidal/columnar lining epithelium is characterized by a light-staining cytoplasm. The intercalated and striated ducts form the duct system **within** the lobular unit, collectively termed the **intralobular** duct system. **Interlobular** ducts are found in the connective tissue between lobules and lined at first by a simple columnar epithelium that becomes pseudostratified and then stratified cuboidal or columnar as the diameter of the duct increases. The surrounding connective tissue also becomes more abundant. **Myoepithelial cells** may be found around the perimeter of the secretory units and initial segments of the duct system. These fibroblast-appearing cells follow the contour of the secretory unit but have a more abundant, light-staining cytoplasm than do fibroblasts. On occasion, cytoplasmic processes can be observed.

The **submandibular gland**, like the parotid, is subdivided into lobes and lobules by connective tissue septa extending from the surrounding capsule. It is a **mixed gland**, with the majority of the secretory units being serous. The **mucous tubules** present usually show **serous demilunes** (crescents) on the blind ends of the secretory tubules that form caps. On occasion, small channels, intercellular secretory canaliculi, can be seen passing between serous and mucous cells and uniting with the lumen of the secretory tubule. Myoepithelial cells also can be observed. Generally, the duct system is similar to that of the parotid, but the **striated ducts** of the intralobular duct system are **much longer** and hence more numerous and conspicuous in sections of the submandibular gland.

The **sublingual gland** also is a **mixed gland** with the majority of secretory units being formed by mucous cells. Serous cells are for the most part organized into demilunes although a few serous tubules will be encountered. Like the other salivary glands myoepithelial are found primarily in relation to the secretory units.

Segments of the **intralobular ducts**, although present, are short and therefore not seen as often in sections of the sublingual as in the other two major salivary glands.

Make a labeled sketch of each of the major salivary glands comparing their histologic features. The sketches should detail the nature of the ductal system and the secretory components.

Teeth

If a ground section of tooth is available, examine it for crown, root, enamel, cementum, dentin and pulp cavity. Determine if the section is from an incisor or molar tooth. Can the cementum be visualized? Under increased magnification, examine the dentin-enamel junction and dentinal tubules, the small tubules coursing through the dentine perpendicular to the pulp cavity.

If a decalcified section through alveolar bone containing a tooth root is available identify the following. Begin in the pulp cavity and note that its circumference is lined by a layer of cells, the **odontoblasts**. Is the surrounding large, darker-staining region of dentine crossed by minute canals, the **dentinal tubules**? Is the **cementum** covering the tooth root cellular or acellular cementum? Can **cementocytes** be observed in **lacunae** of the cementum? Note the thick bundles of collagen fibers that run between the cementum covering the tooth root and the surrounding alveolar bone. This is the **periodontal membrane**. The collagen fibers extend into the bone and cementum as **Sharpey s fibers** to anchor the tooth firmly in the socket of alveolar bone. Note the rich vascular supply associated with the periodontal membrane.

Sketch and label the features observed comparing and contrasting these two types of preparation.

If a routine histologic section of a developing tooth is available examine it for forming enamel and dentin. At low power the developing tooth can be recognized as a V-shaped structure associated with developing alveolar bone. Identify and sketch the following layers seen in a developing tooth. The outermost layer covering the developing tooth consists of tall columnar cells, the **ameloblasts**. Ameloblast apices abut the layer they produce, the **enamel**. Note the position of the nuclei in the layer of ameloblasts. The enamel stains more intensely than any other region of developing tooth and is laid down as a series of prisms. Immediately adjacent to the enamel is the **dentine**, which stains lighter. A region of dentine (predentin) that stains even lighter is found immediately adjacent to the layer of odontoblasts.

Both types of dentine are traversed by thin processes (dentinal fibers) extending from cells of the adjacent odontoblast layer which lie in the minute **dentinal tubules**. **Odontoblasts** produce the dentine and line the interior of the **forming pulp cavity**, which consists of a primitive vascularized mesenchymal tissue.

Sketch and label a developing tooth.

Alimentary canal

The tubular portion of the digestive system consists of four strata, or layers, throughout its length: a mucosa, submucosa, muscularis externa and a serosa or adventitia. The **mucosa** is subdivided into three layers: an **epithelial lining**; its supporting connective tissue, the **lamina propria**; that may contain glands, and a thin smooth muscle layer associated with the mucosa, the **muscularis mucosae**. The **submucosa** is made up of a coarse connective tissue that unites the mucosa to the surrounding muscle wall, the **muscularis externa**. The submucosa is, with two exceptions, aglandular but does contain the larger blood vessels that course around the circumference of the lumen to supply smaller tributaries to the mucosa. An autonomic nerve plexus, the **submucosal** or **Meissner's plexus**, also is found in the submucosa of the alimentary canal throughout its length. These should be identified in each segment of the gut examined. The supporting gut wall, the **muscularis externa**, generally consists of two layers of smooth muscle: an **inner circular layer** and an **outer longitudinal layer**. Examine the connective tissue seam between these two layers of smooth muscle for the second autonomic nerve plexus associated with the gut, the **myenteric** or **Auerbach's plexus**. The latter should be examined in each segment of gut studied. The outermost layer is either a thin connective tissue **adventitia** that binds the tube to surrounding structures or a **serosa,** which consists of a thin layer of connective tissue covered by a mesothelium. The latter is equivalent to the visceral layer of the peritoneum. It should be appreciated that the entire gut tube consists of these basic strata and only the subcomponents differ which are directly related to the function of a given region.

Esophagus

The esophagus is a simple tube that unites the oral cavity to the stomach. Examine a section of esophagus at low power and determine if the section represents a longitudinal or transverse profile as well as which surface is the mucosal surface (contains the lining epithelium).

Beginning at the luminal surface, examine and sketch the **mucosa** noting the very thick, **nonkeratinized stratified squamous epithelium**, the **lamina propria** and a relatively thick **muscularis mucosae**. What is the primary function of the epithelium lining the esophagus? Are glands present within the lamina propria? If so, these compound tubuloalveolar glands represent **esophageal cardiac glands**, which usually are present at the proximal and distal ends of the esophagus. Secretory units are primarily mucous in nature. Examine the connective tissue of the submucosa. Identify larger blood vessels in this layer as well as any profiles of Meissner's plexus. Are compound tubuloalveolar glands present? If so, these are **esophageal proper glands**, found throughout the submucosa of the esophagus. Return to the low-power objective and examine the two thick layers of muscle comprising the **muscularis externa**. Identify the **inner circular** and **outer longitudinal layers**. Determine which region of the esophagus the section was gathered from. If from the upper quarter, the muscularis externa will consist primarily of skeletal muscle; if from the second quarter, a mixture of skeletal and smooth muscle will be encountered; and if from the distal half, it will consist only of smooth muscle. Examine the seam of connective tissue between the inner and outer layers of the muscularis externa for the myenteric plexus. Note the loosely arranged connective tissue of the **adventitia** on the external surface of the esophagus.

Make a sketch illustrating a segment of the esophageal wall and label its subcomponents. The sketch should detail the components of the muscularis externa as well as the perikarya of several neurons and their associated unmyelinated nerve fibers forming the myenteric plexus.

Stomach

Examine several sections of stomach at low power and determine the plane of section, the mucosal surface and the positions of the remaining strata forming the stomach wall.

Examine the simple columnar epithelium lining the luminal surface and note the numerous mucin granules in the apical cytoplasm of each cell. These are unstained in H&E preparations but can be visualized by lowering the condenser and reducing the intensity of light. The surface lining epithelium is organized into simple tubular invaginations called **gastric pits** or **foveolae**. The bottoms of the gastric pits are joined to underlying glands. If the region of the stomach that contains the cardiac glands is examined, note the nearly equal depth of the gastric pits to underlying glands. These are simple tubular or simple branched tubular glands. The **cardiac glands** are organized into lobule-like aggregates by connective tissue elements of the lamina propria and consist primarily of mucous cells with scattered enteroendocrine cells being present. If a section illustrating the esophageal-gastric junction is available, note the very abrupt change from the thick non-keratinized stratified squamous epithelium lining the esophagus to the simple columnar epithelium lining the stomach.

Sections from the **body** and **fundic** regions of the stomach contain much longer oxyntic (fundic) glands as compared to other regions of the stomach. Note in this case that the ratio of depth of the gastric pit to depth of the oxyntic gland is about 1:4. Next, examine the cellular components of the simple branched tubular **oxyntic glands**, which consist of four cell types: mucous neck cells, parietal cells, chief cells and enteroendocrine cells. **Mucous neck cells** are most numerous in the neck region of the gastric glands (that region that joins the bottom of a gastric pit) but are scattered for variable distances deep within the oxyntic glands. Mucous neck cells are small, show a variable morphology and contain numerous mucin granules that remain unstained in H&E preparations. The granules often exhibit an empty or frothy appearance. These cells may show a wide apex and a narrow base or a wide base and a narrow apex and are sandwiched between other cell types. **Parietal cells** are large, round cells that appear to bulge out and away from their associated oxyntic glands. The cells stain a light red-orange and often exhibit a granular appearance. The eosinophilia and granular appearance is due to the numerous mitochondria associated with parietal cells which stain with the eosin dye and result in the red-orange granular appearance. Parietal cells are abundant and scattered throughout the length of the oxyntic glands but are seen with greater frequency in the upper half of the gland. In contrast, **chief (zymogen) cells** are confined primarily to the bases of the oxyntic glands. These cells are pyramidal in shape, have a light basophilic cytoplasm and large, homogeneous apical cytoplasmic granules. Scattered between the bases of chief and parietal cells near the bottoms of the oxyntic glands are small oval or round cells with a light (clear)-appearing cytoplasm and central nuclei. Tiny dust-like secretory granules may be present in the basal cytoplasm. These are the **enteroendocrine (endocrine) cells**.

The pylorus or pyloric region of the stomach contains **pyloric glands**. These are simple branched tubular glands whose primary cellular component are mucous cells. The depth ratio of pit to gland like that of the cardiac gland region is about 1:1.

Enteroendocrine cells also are present in considerable numbers and parietal cells can be found scattered within these glands particularly near the junction with the body of the stomach. Note the scant, delicate connective tissue of the lamina propria around all three types of glands. Plasma cells, mast cells and lymphocytes are commonly found in the lamina propria of the stomach. Carefully examine the well-defined **muscularis mucosae** (located immediately beneath the glands) and its subcomponents (inner circular, outer longitudinal layers). Note that slips of smooth muscle extend from the muscularis mucosae to enter the lamina propria and course toward the mucosal surface.

Sketch in detail the gastric mucosa representative of all three glandular regions. Detail the relationships of glands to overlying gastric pits as well as the type and location of component cells.

Examine the details of the **submucosa**. This is a coarse connective tissue layer with large caliber interwoven collagen fibers and scattered mast and lymphoid cells. The submucosa also houses small arteries, veins and lymphatic vessels. Elements of **Meissner s plexus** also will be encountered.

Make a sketch of each of these structures and their position within the submucosa.

Examine the thick **muscularis externa** and its inner circular and outer longitudinal layers. Some regions (primarily the fundus) may also exhibit an inner oblique layer. As with the esophagus, examine the connective tissue seam between the two layers of the muscularis externa for elements of **Auerbach s (myenteric) plexus**. If the junction between the stomach and small intestine is available, examine the large expansion of the inner circular component of the muscularis externa, which forms the **pyloric sphincter**.

The outermost layer of the stomach wall is the **serosa**. It consists of a thin connective tissue layer adhering to the outer limit of the muscularis externa and is covered by a simple squamous epithelium (mesothelium). This layer is the histological equivalent to the visceral layer of the peritoneum.

Small intestine

The small intestine is subdivided into three macroscopic regions: duodenum, jejunum and ileum. All show the same basic organization, although there are minor microscopic differences among subdivisions. Determine the mucosal surface, which will stain a deeper blue because of the greater concentration of nuclei per unit area. Next examine the different segments of the small intestine under low power and identify the four basic strata. Examine the section for large folds characterized by a core of submucosa. These large macroscopic folds, the **plicae circulares**, can be seen with the naked eye if the slide is held up to the light and viewed directly. Note that the intestinal mucosa is in the form of numerous finger-like evaginations called villi. **Villi** consist of a **lamina propria core** and a **covering of intestinal epithelium**. Villi measure 0.5 - 1.5 mm in length and are larger in the duodenum and jejunum than in the ileum, where they generally become shorter and more finger-like. Simple tubular **intestinal glands (crypts of Lieberk hn)** extend from between the bases of the villi and into the lamina propria. The intestinal glands measure 0.3 - 0.5 mm in depth and extend through the lamina propria to the level of the muscularis mucosae. The glands are separated from one another by the very cellular reticular connective tissue of the lamina propria. Re-examine the lamina propria and fully appreciate that it is continuous, ie, fills the cores of villi and the areas between and around the intestinal glands. The lamina propria is rich in reticular fibers that support numerous lymphocytes, plasma cells, macrophages and eosinophils, giving the lamina propria its very cellular appearance. The lamina propria of the intestinal tract represents a special type of lymphatic tissue and is part of the **gut associated lymphatic tissue** or GALT. Lymphatic nodules of variable size lie in the lamina propria scattered along the entire length of intestinal tract but become more numerous and larger distally. They are particularly numerous and well developed in the ileum. Here the lymphatic nodules may occur singly or grouped together in aggregates called **Peyer s patches**. These oval structures may be quite large (~ 20mm in length) and are visible to the naked eye. They may occupy the full depths of both the mucosa and submucosa.

Note that the **muscularis mucosae** is well defined but thin when compared to that of the esophagus and stomach. It consists of inner circular and outer longitudinal layers. Closely examine the muscularis mucosae with the high-power objective. Identify slips of smooth muscle that leave the muscularis mucosae and enter the cores of villi to provide a means by which villi contract. Note too that small arteries are present on the inner surface of the muscularis mucosae. These subdivide into an extensive **capillary network** that lies just beneath the intestinal epithelium covering the villi. Examine the interior (center) of the lamina propria core within villi for the presence of an endothelium lined elongated space. These do not contain erythrocytes and represent the start of lymphatic channels called **central lacteals**.

Make sketches illustrating the relationship of villi and intestinal glands to the lamina propria. Illustrate a lymphatic nodule in the lamina propria as well as the position of the capillary plexus and the central lacteal.

Return to the luminal surface and carefully examine the simple columnar intestinal epithelium. Note that unlike the homogeneous simple columnar epithelium that lines the stomach, that lining the intestinal tract consists of a heterogeneous population of cells. The most numerous epithelial cell type is the **enterocyte** or **absorptive intestinal cell**. It is a tall, cylindrical cell and shows a prominent **striated (microvillus) border** at its free surface. With the high-power objective carefully examine the striated border. Look for minute intense rods occurring between apices of adjacent intestinal epithelial cells. These are terminal bars. **Goblet cells** occur scattered between intestinal absorptive cells and increase in number distally in the intestinal tract. Confirm that the apical regions of goblet cells are often expanded by an accumulation of unstained secretory granules; the base forms a slender region that contains the nucleus. **Enteroendocrine (endocrine) cells** are also present in the intestinal epithelium of both villi and intestinal glands but are fewer in number than goblet cells. They often exhibit a clear or light-staining cytoplasm and may be spindle-shaped, extending from the luminal surface to the basal surface of the intestinal epithelium. Others appear as small oval or dome-shaped cells within the basal region of the intestinal epithelium. Both forms often show tiny dust-like granules in the basal cytoplasm. Small groups of pyramidal-shaped cells with conspicuous, large eosinophilic granules in the apical cytoplasm are found at the bottoms of the intestinal glands. These are **Paneth cells**. Identify **intraepithelial lymphocytes** found within and between intestinal epithelial cells covering villi and forming intestinal glands. Note the numerous **mitotic figures within the intestinal glands**.

Make a detailed sketch of each of the cell types encountered and their position within the intestinal epithelium covering the villi or forming the intestinal glands.

Examine the connective tissue of the submucosa and look for large arteries, veins, lymphatics and elements of **Meissner s plexus**. The duodenum is characterized by the presence of branched tubular glands of the mucous type in the submucosa. The ducts of these **duodenal glands (Brunner s glands)** pierce the muscularis mucosae and empty, most often, into the bottoms of overlying intestinal glands.

Make a sketch of these glands and illustrate their position within the duodenal wall.

Examine the **muscularis externa** of the various segments along the small intestine. It consists of inner circular and outer longitudinal layers of smooth muscle. Look for and identify elements of **Auerbach s plexus** in the connective tissue seam between these two muscle layers. Examine the external surface of the duodenum for an **adventitia**. Examine the external surface of the ileum for a **serosa**. How can the difference between the adventitia and serosa be determined? What morphologic features can be used to differentiate sections of duodenum, jejunum and ileum? Because the mucosa of the duodenum and jejunum is very similar, the major histological feature that differentiates these two segments of the small intestine is the **presence** or **absence** of the **duodenal glands**. Regions of the ileum contain substantially more goblet cells than either the duodenum or jejunum. Examine all three regions quickly at low power for a comparison of the number of goblet cells.

Colon

Examine a region of the colon. Note, using the low-power objective, that it resembles the wall of the small intestine with **two notable exceptions:** the colon **lacks villi** and the outer longitudinal layer of the muscularis externa is gathered into **three taenia coli**. View the colon under high power and confirm that the lumen of the colon is lined by a simple columnar epithelium that consists primarily of intestinal absorptive cells (enterocytes) and goblet cells. Goblet cells increase in number toward the rectum so that in distal regions the epithelium consists primarily of goblet cells. Note that the intestinal glands are longer and more closely packed than those of the small intestine. The glands contain numerous goblet cells and mitotic figures are encountered in the basal half of these glands. Observe that the composition of the lamina propria and muscularis mucosae is the same as that found in the small intestine, as is the submucosa. As observed earlier, the outer, longitudinal layer of the muscularis externa of the colon is formed into three longitudinal bands called taeniae coli. Between the taeniae this layer of smooth muscle is quite thin and may be incomplete. The inner circular layer of the muscularis externa is complete and appears similar to that of the small intestine. The **myenteric plexus** lies just external to the inner circular layer. Dependent on which segment of the colon is being examined a serosa or adventitia may be observed. Ascending and descending limbs of the colon are retroperitoneal, hence are covered by an **adventitia**.

Where a **serosa** is present, large lobules of fat called **appendices epiploicae** may be encountered.

Sketch a region of colon and label its subcomponents.

Appendix

Using low power, observe that the morphologic features of a section of appendix resembles those of the colon but **in miniature**. The lumen is small and irregular in shape and the taeniae coli are absent. The lamina propria is highly infiltrated with lymphocytes and lymphatic nodules may fill the mucosa and submucosa.

Primary junctions between segments of the alimentary canal

The **esophageal-gastric junction** is characterized by dramatic changes in the mucosa. The thick, non-keratinized stratified squamous epithelium of the esophagus changes abruptly to a tall simple columnar epithelium lining the stomach. The gastric mucosa also exhibits gastric pits and underlying simple branched tubular cardiac glands consisting primarily of mucous cells.

At the **gastrointestinal junction** the homogeneous simple columnar epithelium lining the stomach changes **abruptly** to a simple columnar epithelium of the intestine composed of a heterogeneous population of cells. Note the **microvillus border on enterocytes** and scattered **goblet cells**. In the stomach note the **gastric pits** and the **pyloric glands** joining their bases. **Both lie in the mucosa** on the luminal side of the muscularis mucosae. As the gastrointestinal junction is crossed, note the change in epithelial lining as well as the position of associated glands. On the intestinal (duodenal) side of the junction, **the duodenal glands (of Brunner) lie in the submucosa below the level of the muscularis mucosae**. Note the expansion of the inner circular layer of the muscularis externa immediately proximal to these changes to form the **pyloric sphincter**.

Observe that at the **rectoanal junction** an abrupt change from the simple columnar intestinal epithelium (with goblet cells) lining the rectum to the nonkeratinized stratified squamous epithelium of the anal canal. Note also that the intestinal glands and muscularis mucosae of the rectum **disappear** at the rectoanal junction. Next examine and trace elements of the muscularis externa. The inner circular layer of the muscularis externa increases in thickness and ends as the **internal anal sphincter**. The outer longitudinal layer of smooth muscle breaks up and ends in the surrounding connective tissue. **Skeletal muscle fibers** encircle the distal anal canal and form the **external anal sphincter**.

Sketch the primary junctions between segments of the alimentary canal comparing and contrasting changes in structure.

Table 12. Key histologic features of the alimentary tract (Esophagus and Stomach).

Region	Epithelium	Muscularis mucosae	Muscularis externa	Lymphatic tissue	Glands
Esophagus	Nonkeratinized stratified squamous	Prominent inner circular and outer longitudinal layers of smooth muscle	Outer longitudinal, inner circular layers. Skeletal muscle upper one-quarter, mixed smooth and skeletal middle one-quarter, smooth muscle in lower half	Occasional nodules, diffuse in lamina propria	1. Esophageal proper, scattered along length of esophagus in submucosa, compound tubuloalveolar mucus-secreting 2. Esophageal cardiac, proximal and distal ends in lamina propria; compound tubuloalveolar, mucus-secreting
Stomach Cardia	Simple columnar	Smooth muscle; outer longitudinal; inner circular, a third outer circular layer in some areas	Smooth muscle, outer longitudinal, middle circular, inner oblique layer	Small patches of diffuse lymphatic tissue; occasional nodules	Long gastric pits (one-half the depth of mucosa); simple branched tubular; mucous, endocrine, and occasional parietal cells
Fundus and Body	Simple columnar	Same	Same	Same	Short gastric pits (one-fourth the depth of the mucosa); simple branched tubular; mucous neck, parietal, chief, and endocrine cells
Pylorus	Simple columnar	Smooth muscle; outer longitudinal, inner circular	Same	Occasional small lymphatic nodules in lamina propria	Long gastric pits (one-half the depth of mucosa); simple branched tubular; mucous, occasional parietal and numerous endocrine cells

Table 13. Key histologic features of the alimentary tract (Intestinal tract and Anal canal).

Region	Epithelium	Muscularis mucosae	Muscularis externa	Lymphatic tissue	Glands
Duodenum	Villi covered by enterocytes with microvillus border; goblet and endocrine cells	Inner circular, outer longitudinal layers of smooth muscle	Inner circular, outer longitudinal layers of smooth muscle; myenteric plexus between layers	Solitary nodules and diffuse lymphatic tissue	1. Simple tubular intestinal glands in lamina propria; goblet, endocrine, and Paneth cells 2. Brunner s glands in submucosa
Remainder of small intestine	Villi covered by enterocytes; goblet cells increase in number distally; endocrine cells present	Same	Same	Nodular lymphatic tissue forms aggregates (Peyer s patches) in ileum	Intestinal glands; same as for duodenum
Colon	Villi absent; lumen lined by enterocytes; goblet cells increased in number	Same	Outer longitudinal layer organized into 3 bands: taeniae coli	Solitary nodules and diffuse lymphatic tissue	Intestinal glands; absorptive, goblet, and endocrine cells
Rectum	Enterocytes; mainly goblet cells	Same	Inner circular and outer longitudinal layers	Solitary nodules	Intestinal glands; goblet cells more abundant
Anal canal	At pectinate line becomes wet stratified squamous, then cornified at orifice	Disappears at level of anal columns	Inner circular layer of smooth muscle thickens to form internal anal sphincter; outer longitudinal layer disappears replaced by skeletal muscle of external anal sphincter	Solitary nodules	1. Intestinal glands disappear at pectinate line 2. Apocrine sweat glands appear associated with thin skin

Pancreas

The pancreas is covered by a thin connective tissue capsule from which delicate septa extend and subdivide it into numerous small lobules. The parenchyma consists of an exocrine portion and an endocrine portion, each consisting of a different group of cells.

Learning objectives for the pancreas:

1. Be able to distinguish between the exocrine and endocrine regions of the pancreas and be able to recognize the subcomponents of each.

The **exocrine pancreas** is a large **compound tubuloacinar (alveolar) gland** the secretory units of which consist of **large pyramidal serous (acinar) cells** whose narrow apices border a tiny lumen. Observe that the apical cytoplasm is filled with large **secretory (zymogen) granules** and that the basal cytoplasm stains basophilic due to the intense concentration of granular endoplasmic reticulum. The ductal system is extensive and permeates the pancreas. The ductal system **begins** within the interior of the secretory units **as centroacinar cells**. Component cells appear flattened and are light staining. These are continuous outside the secretory unit with **intercalated** and **intralobular ducts**. These are tributaries of larger interlobular ducts found in the loose connective tissue between lobules. The transition between ducts is gradual with the epithelium beginning as simple squamous in the intercalated ducts, increases in height to cuboidal in intralobular ducts, and is columnar in the **interlobular ducts**. A delicate connective tissue consisting primarily of reticular fibers surrounds the intralobular ducts. The interlobular ducts and main secretory ducts lie within interlobular septa and are therefore enveloped by a larger amount of connective tissue.

The **endocrine pancreas** consists of irregular elongated masses of pale-staining cells called the **pancreatic islets** or **islets of Langerhans** scattered between elements of the exocrine pancreas. The islets are separated from the exocrine pancreas by a delicate investment of reticular fibers that contains numerous capillaries. In typical H&E sections the islets appear to be composed of a homogeneous population of pale-staining cells, but with special stains and immunohistochemistry, four distinct cell types can be demonstrated. **Beta (insulin-containing) cells** form about 78% of the islet cells and tend to be near the center of the islet. **Alpha (glucagon-containing) cells** make up about 20% of the islets and are generally located at the periphery of the islet. **Delta** (somatostatin-containing) **cells** and **PP (pancreatic polypeptide-containing) cells** also are present in small numbers at the periphery of the islets. All four endocrine cell types can be found, on occasion, scattered individually within the ducts and acini of the exocrine pancreas where they form a small population.

Make a labeled sketch of the pancreas illustrating both exocrine and endocrine components.

Liver

The liver, like the pancreas, is both an exocrine and endocrine gland secreting bile into a duct system and releasing several substances directly into the blood stream. Unlike the pancreas, however, the liver cells or **hepatocytes** perform both functions.

Learning objectives for the liver:

1. Be able to identify several classic hepatic lobules and their subcomponents.
2. Be able to relate the flow of blood and bile to the morphology of a hepatic lobule.
3. Be able to identify portal areas and their contents as well as distinguish the layers that form the wall of the gall bladder.

The liver is invested by a delicate connective tissue **capsule** rich in elastic fibers and covered by a mesothelium except for a small area where the liver abuts the diaphragm. Hepatocytes are arranged in branching, anastomosing plates separated by blood sinusoids both of which form a radial pattern about a central vein. The spokelike arrangement of hepatic plates about a central vein constitutes the basis of the **classic hepatic lobule**. The liver consists of about 1 million of such repeating units, each about 2.0 mm long and 0.7 mm wide.

Using the low power objective identify several of these hexagonal units as seen in transverse section. Note the position of the **central vein** at the center, the radiating plates of hepatocytes separated by **sinusoids**, and **portal areas** in a small amount of connective tissue at the corners of the lobules.

Sketch and label the contents of three adjacent hepatic lobules.

Each portal area contains a small branch of the **hepatic artery**, a branch of the **portal vein**, a **bile duct** and on occasion a **lymphatic channel**.

Be aware that blood passes from these branches of the hepatic artery and portal vein into the sinusoids that lie between the hepatic plates. Blood then flows slowly through the sinusoids toward the center of the lobule to exit through the central vein, which is the smallest tributary of the hepatic vein. Now examine each of the structural elements at increased magnification.

Beginning with the **hepatic sinusoids** note that they are larger and more irregular in shape than ordinary capillaries. The sinusoidal lining consists of a simple squamous **endothelium** supported by very little connective tissue. Two additional cell types are associated with the sinusoidal lining: **hepatic macrophages (Kupffer cells)** and **fat-storing cells (lipocytes)**. Both can be demonstrated using special preparations but usually are difficult to differentiate in routine preparations. Note that the sinusoidal lining is separated from the hepatocytes by a narrow **perisinusoidal space**. Hepatocytes are large and polyhedral in shape, and exhibit large, round nuclei that usually occupy the center of the cell. A single nucleus of variable size is usually present, however as many as 25% of hepatocytes are binucleate. The cytoplasm is variable in appearance and changes with the nutritive state of the liver. **Bile canaliculi**, tiny channels that course through the parenchyma between hepatocytes, end in the **interlobular bile ducts** of the portal areas. Look carefully between adjacent hepatocytes using the high-power objective for minute circular or elongated spaces-these are bile canaliculi.

Examine a portal area at increased magnification and note that the **hepatic artery** is in actual fact an arteriole with only one or two layers of smooth muscle. The **portal vein** can be identified as a collapsed thin-walled endothelium-lined space that usually contains erythrocytes and/or plasma. Similar structures devoid of red blood cells and plasma may indeed be **lymphatic channels**. The **bile duct** is usually lined by a simple cuboidal epithelium surrounded by a scant connective tissue. As the bile ducts course toward the exterior, the lumina increase in diameter, the epithelium increases in height and the surrounding layers of connective tissue become thicker.

Carefully examine and sketch the contents of a portal area.

Gallbladder

The gallbladder is a sac-like structure measuring about 8 cm long and 4 cm wide located on the inferior surface of the liver. It consists of a mucosa, a muscularis, and an adventitia. The **mucosa** consists of a simple, tall columnar epithelium supported by an underlying lamina propria of delicate connective tissue. Note the elaborately folded nature of the mucosa. The **muscularis** consists of interlacing bundles of smooth muscle the gaps between bundles of which are filled with collagenous, reticular and elastic fibers. An **adventitia** of fibroelastic connective tissue is fairly thick and at the free surface (that facing the abdominal cavity) is covered by mesothelium forming a **serosa**.

Make a sketch detailing the structure of the gallbladder wall.

The respiratory system consists of conducting and respiratory portions. The conducting portion delivers air to the respiratory portion in the lungs and consists of nasal cavities, pharynx, larynx, trachea and various subdivisions of the bronchial tree. The respiratory portion is where gaseous exchange takes place.

Learning objectives for the respiratory system:

1. Be able to distinguish the various regions and subdivisions of the respiratory system.

Nose

Skin covers the external surface of the nose and extends for a short distance into the vestibule of the nasal cavity. Here, large hairs and their associated sebaceous glands are found. Note that more posteriorly, the vestibule is lined by nonkeratinized stratified squamous epithelium. The remainder of the nasal cavity is lined by a **ciliated pseudostratified columnar epithelium with goblet cells**; however, a specialized olfactory epithelium is present in the roof of the nasal cavities. A layer of delicate connective tissue, the **lamina propria**, underlies the epithelium and contains mucous and serous glands as well as thin-walled venous sinuses. **Venous sinuses** are especially prominent in the lamina propria covering the middle and inferior conchae. The deep layers of the lamina propria merge with the periosteum or perichondrium of the nasal bones and cartilages, and at these sites the nasal mucosa is referred to as a **mucoperiosteum** or **mucoperichondrium**, respectively. **Paranasal sinuses** lie within bones (maxillary, sphenoid, frontal, ethmoid) surrounding the nasal cavity and are continuous with it through small openings. The lining epithelium of the paranasal sinuses is the same and continuous with that lining the remainder of the nasal cavity in this region.

Olfactory epithelium

The olfactory epithelium lines the roof of the nasal cavity where it extends over the superior conchae and for a short distance on either side of the nasal septum. It is a **thick pseudostratified columnar epithelium** that **lacks goblet cells**. Olfactory epithelium consists primarily of three different cell types: supporting cells, basal cells and sensory (olfactory) cells. The **supporting (sustentacular) cells** are tall columnar with narrow bases and broad apical surfaces. An oval nucleus is located near the center of the cell. Sensory cells are in fact **bipolar nerve cells** evenly distributed among supporting cells. Sensory cells are spindle-

shaped with round nuclei located in a central expanded region of the cytoplasm. A single slender process (a modified dendrite) extends apically between supporting cells and at the surface expands to form a bulblike **olfactory vesicle (knob)**. Six to eight long **olfactory cilia** extend from the olfactory vesicle and lie parallel to the surface of the olfactory epithelium. A thin process, an **axon**, extends from the base of these cells into the underlying lamina propria, where, with similar axons, it forms small nerve bundles called **fila olfactoria**. In addition to the mature form of bipolar nerve cell, numerous stages of differentiating bipolar olfactory neurons are present in this unique sensory epithelium. These eventually replace the mature form, the life span of which is between 30 and 60 days. **Basal cells** are short, pyramidal cells that lie on the basement membrane crowded between the bases of the sustentacular and sensory cells. Carefully examine the olfactory epithelium for all three cell types. Why is the olfactory epithelium so thick?

Examine the connective tissue forming the lamina propria and identify several examples of venous sinuses, fila olfactoria as well as the **olfactory (Bowman's) glands**. The latter are branched, tubuloacinar serous glands.

Make a detailed, labeled sketch of the olfactory epithelium together with associated structures found in the underlying lamina propria.

Nasopharynx

The nasal cavities continue posteriorly into the nasopharynx, which is lined by the same respiratory passage epithelium found in the nasal cavities, ie, ciliated pseudostratified columnar epithelium with goblet cells. The underlying lamina propria contains mucous, serous and mixed mucoserous glands and abundant lymphatic tissue. The remainder of the pharynx is lined by nonkeratinized stratified squamous epithelium.

Larynx

The larynx connects the pharynx and trachea. Its supporting framework consists of several cartilages, of which the thyroid, cricoid and arytenoids are hyaline, while the epiglottis, corniculates and tips of the arytenoids are elastic. The cartilages are united by sheets of dense collagenous connective tissue. The epithelial lining varies with location. The anterior surface and about half the posterior surface of the epiglottis are covered by nonkeratinized stratified squamous epithelium.

The epithelium of these regions may contain scattered taste buds. The vocal cords also are covered by non-keratinized stratified squamous epithelium. The remainder of the larynx is lined by typical respiratory passage-type epithelium. The lamina propria of the larynx is thick and contains mucous and some serous or mucoserous glands.

Trachea and extrapulmonary bronchi

The walls of the trachea and primary bronchi are characterized by the presence of **C-shaped rings of hyaline cartilage**. These can be seen by direct visual examination of the slide. The area between **successive** rings is filled with dense fibroelastic connective tissue. Note using the low-power objective that the gaps between the arms of the cartilages are linked by bundles of smooth muscle. This is the trachealis muscle. The epithelial lining of the trachea and extrapulmonary bronchi consists of **ciliated pseudostratified columnar epithelium** with numerous **goblet cells** and rests on a thick basement membrane. Identify **short cells** that occur in the depths of the epithelium between the bases of the other two cell types. The underlying submucosa contains numerous seromucous (tracheal) glands and occasional accumulations of lymphatic tissue. Examine the connective tissue forming the **adventitia** that covers the external surface of the trachea for small blood vessels and nerves.

Make a labeled sketch of a transverse section through the trachea.

Table 14. Key histologic features of the respiratory system.				
Division	**Part**	**Epithelium**	**Support**	**Other features**
Extrapulmonary conducting	Main portion of nasal cavity	Ciliated pseudostratified columnar with goblet cells (respiratory epithelium)	Hyaline cartilage and bone	Lamina propria forms a mucoperiosteum; contains seromucous glands and large venous sinuses
	Olfactory region of nasal cavity	Thick pseudostratified columnar with 3 cell types: Olfactory bipolar neurons, sustentacular cells, basal cells	Bone of nasal conchae and septum	Lamina propria forms mucoperiosteum; contains serous glands, venous sinuses and nerves
	Nasopharynx	Respiratory lining epithelium	Skeletal muscle	Lamina propria contains mucous, serous and mucoserous glands; abundant lymphatic tissue; pharyngeal tonsils
	Oral pharynx	Nonkeratinized stratified squamous	Skeletal muscle	As above; palatine tonsils
	Laryngeal area	Nonkeratinized stratified squamous to middle posterior surface of epiglottis and over vocal cords; respiratory lining epithelium elsewhere	Cartilage; dense regular connective tissue	Epiglottis, corniculate cartilage, tips of arytenoid are elastic cartilage, other laryngeal cartilages are hyaline; taste buds may occur in epithelium covering epiglottis
	Trachea and main bronchi	Respiratory lining epithelium	C-shaped hyaline cartilages; fibro-elastic connective tissue between	Lamina propria separated from submucosa by elastic tissue; seromucous (tracheal) glands in submucosa; scattered lymphatic tissue

Intrapulmonary conducting units

Scan a section of lung with the low-power objective noting the position of several circular or tubular structures with a distinct limiting wall. Observe that some are larger and appear more prominent than others. These are segments of the intrapulmonary conducting system. Beginning with the largest, examine the histologic features of the limiting wall starting at the luminal surface. Having completed this exercise return to low power and find a slightly smaller segment and examine it at increased magnification. In this way systematically examine all the tubular units in the section of lung proceeding from the largest to the smallest detailing the structural composition of the wall forming each unit.

Recall that the primary bronchi divide and give rise to several orders of intrapulmonary bronchi. In these structures a supporting framework of irregular shaped plates of hyaline cartilage completely surrounds the lumen. Note that the lumen continues to be lined by a **ciliated pseudostratified columnar epithelium** with **goblet cells** that rest on a basement membrane. The underlying lamina propria may contain diffuse lymphatic tissue. A thin smooth muscle layer is now apparent and separates the lamina propria from the connective tissue of the **submucosa**, which lies immediately internal to the plates of cartilage. Mucous and mucoserous **bronchial glands** are present in the submucosa. Note that their ducts penetrate the muscle layer to open onto the epithelial surface. The smallest of the intrapulmonary bronchi show only isolated cartilage plates and the epithelium changes to a **ciliated simple columnar** with **goblet cells**. Bronchial glands extend as far down the respiratory tree as do the cartilages plates. As the diameter of the bronchial tree reaches about 1 mm, cartilage disappears from the wall and the structure is termed a **bronchiole**. At this point of transition, the bronchial glands and lymphatic tissue also disappear, however, the bronchial smooth muscle remains fairly prominent and becomes the major supporting element of the bronchiole wall. The lining epithelium varies from ciliated simple columnar with goblet cells in large bronchioles to **ciliated simple cuboidal** with **no goblet cells** in **terminal bronchioles** (the smallest units of the purely conducting system). Scattered among the ciliated cells are a few non-ciliated cells whose apical surfaces bulge into the lumen. These are the **bronchiolar secretory (Clara) cells**, which contain antiproteases and oxidases. They have also been implicated in surfactant production.

Make a detailed sketch of several profiles observed during the examination of the intrapulmonary conducting units. Note in particular the changes that have occurred when comparing the largest to the smallest units.

Respiratory tissue

Return to the low-power objective and scan the section of lung again observing its lacy, sponge-like architecture. Observe that in addition to the scattered profiles of the intrapulmonary conducting units, additional elongated spaces can be observed within the lacy tissue comprising the remainder of the lung. Examine these structures more carefully as many represent respiratory bronchioles and alveolar ducts of the respiratory portion of the lung.

Recall that the first region where gaseous exchange takes place is in the **respiratory bronchioles,** which represent a short transition point between the purely conducting and purely respiratory portions of the lung. Its wall consists of collagenous connective tissue with thin interlacing bundles of smooth muscle and elastic fibers. Larger respiratory bronchioles are lined by a ciliated simple cuboidal epithelium with scattered Clara cells. In smaller respiratory bronchioles the epithelium becomes low cuboidal without cilia. In these thin walled transitional units, **alveoli** balloon out from the walls of the respiratory bronchioles and function as the respiratory portions of these airways. In a few places along its length, small groups of cuboidal cells may intervene between successive alveoli and cover an underlying small, narrow bundle of smooth muscle. Respiratory bronchioles end by branching into alveolar ducts. **Alveolar ducts** appear as thin-walled tubes, the walls of which are formed largely by a succession of alveolar openings around its circumference. Alveolar ducts terminate as **alveolar sacs,** which are irregular spaces formed by clusters of alveoli. **Alveoli** are thin-walled, cup-shaped structures that are open at one side to allow air to enter into their cavities. Due to the plane of section many will appear as small circular spaces surrounded by a very thin rim of tissue. Adjacent alveoli are separated by a common interalveolar septum. The most conspicuous feature of the alveolar wall is a rich capillary network that bulges the limiting wall into the alveolar lumen. Note that profiles of erythrocytes within these capillaries can often be made out in the alveolar wall. The majority of the alveolar wall is lined by attenuated simple squamous cells called **pulmonary epithelial cells** or **type I pneumocytes**. Scattered within this epithelial lining are cuboidal cells that often bulge into the alveolar lumen. These are **type II pneumocytes** which are further characterized by numerous small, light-staining vacuoles in their cytoplasm. It is this cell type that produces alveolar surfactant.

On occasion, **alveolar macrophages** (dust cells) may be observed in either the alveolar wall or lumen which usually contain phagocytosed particles of inhaled material.

The external surface of the lung is covered by **visceral pleura** which consists of collagenous and elastic fibers covered by a single layer of mesothelial cells.

Make a labeled sketch illustrating the transition from respiratory bronchiole to alveolar duct to a cluster of alveoli. Note in particular the changes that occur in the lining epithelium as well as those of the supporting wall.

Make an additional sketch of adjacent alveoli illustrating an alveolar septum and the epithelial cells lining the alveoli. Compare the light microscopic observations with those seen using the electron microscope.

Table 15. Key histologic features of the respiratory system.

Division	Part	Epithelium	Supporting wall	Other features
Intrapulmonary conducting	Intrapulmonary bronchi	Respiratory epithelium in the largest; ciliated simple columnar with goblet cells in the smallest	Irregular, discontinuous plates of hyaline cartilage decreasing in smaller bronchi	Smooth muscle increasingly prominent as cartilage disappears; mucoserous glands and lymphatic tissue in submucosa
Intrapulmonary conducting	Bronchioles	Ciliated simple columnar with goblet cells in the largest to ciliated columnar without goblet cells in the smallest	Smooth muscle	Connective tissue decreased in amount; no glands or lymphatic tissue present
Transition from conducting to respiratory portions	Respiratory bronchioles	Simple cuboidal, some ciliated, no goblet cells; Clara cells present	Thin layer of fibroelastic connective tissue; few smooth muscle cells	Alveoli bud out from wall
Respiratory portion	Alveolar ducts	Cuboidal, nonciliated epithelial cells between successive alveoli	Thin, delicate connective tissue	Tubular shaped wall formed in part by successive alveoli
Respiratory portion	Alveolar sacs	Type I and II pneumocytes, macrophages	Elastic and reticular fibers	Formed by clusters of alveoli
Respiratory portion	Alveoli	Type I and II pneumocytes, macrophages	Elastic and reticular fibers	Blood air barrier consists of cytoplasm of type I pneumocyte, common basement membrane, cytoplasm of endothelial cells

The urinary system consists of the kidneys, ureters, urinary bladder and urethra.

Learning objectives for the urinary system:

1. Be able to distinguish the different regions of a uriniferous tubule and know their location within a section of kidney.
2. Be able to distinguish the different segments of individual nephron units and their subcomponents.
3. Be able to distinguish the collecting tubules (ducts) in the cortex and medulla.
4. Be able to distinguish the various segments of the vascular supply in a section of kidney.
5. Be able to distinguish the different regions of the extrarenal passages and the subcomponents of the three strata forming their limiting walls.

Kidneys

Examination of a section of kidney, either directly or under low power, will determine whether or not the section is of cortex, medulla or contains regions of both. The cortex generally is darker-staining and component tubules are arranged at random. In contrast, the medulla is light-staining and the tubules arranged parallel to one another. Begin by examining the external region of the cortex. Is a connective tissue capsule present on its external surface? Examine the parenchyma of the cortex at low or medium power slowly scanning a large area. Note the abundance of several large circular appearing structures scattered between granular, dark-staining tubules seen in various planes of section. The former are the renal corpuscles, the latter proximal convoluted tubules. **Both are found ONLY in the cortex** and thus can be used in determining which region of the kidney (cortex or medulla) is being viewed.

Return to a **renal corpuscle** and examine it at high power for several histologic features. The renal corpuscle is the first portion of a nephron. It is roughly spherical in shape and measures 150 - 250 μm in diameter. The renal corpuscle consists of two parts: a central capillary tuft, the **glomerulus**, and a surrounding **glomerular (Bowman's) capsule**. This capsule is made up of two layers. The outer layer of the capsule surrounds the glomerulus as the **parietal layer (capsular epithelium)**, which then reflects onto glomerular capillaries as the **visceral layer (glomerular epithelium)**. The visceral and parietal layers of Bowman's capsule are separated by a **capsular space**. Examine the parietal layer and observe that it is a simple squamous epithelium lying on a distinct basement membrane. Scan several renal corpuscles at low power looking for a region known as the vascular pole. The **vascular pole** is that area of the renal corpuscle where the afferent and efferent arterioles join the glomerular capillaries. Examine a vascular pole carefully and note where the simple squamous epithelium of the parietal layer reflects onto the glomerular capillaries. Here, the epithelium changes to a specialized cell type called the **podocyte**. Realize that the podocytes form the glomerular epithelium (visceral layer of Bowman's capsule). Podocytes can be distinguished by their large, light-staining more euchromatic nuclei and relatively abundant cytoplasm. In contrast, glomerular **endothelial cells** exhibit dark-staining, heterochromatic nuclei and a thin attenuated cytoplasm. These two cell types form the glomerular capillary wall and are separated by a **common basement membrane** measuring 0.1 - 0.5 μm in thickness. Continue to examine renal corpuscles for a region known as the **urinary pole**, that region continuous with the second portion of the nephron, the proximal convoluted tubule. At this pole examine the abrupt change in epithelium from simple squamous of the parietal layer to a single layer of large pyramidal-shaped cells forming the proximal convoluted tubule. Note that the capsular space is continuous with the lumen of the proximal convoluted tubule.

The **proximal convoluted tubule** begins at the urinary pole of the renal corpuscle and is the longest segment of the nephron measuring about 17 mm in length. For this reason it is the most commonly observed structure seen in the renal cortex. The proximal tubule is characterized by a stellate shaped lumen and component cells appear more granular and stain more intensely than other structures in the cortex. The proximal convoluted tubule is formed by a single layer of large, pyramidal-shaped cells that have a **well-developed brush (microvillus) border**, which circumscribes the lumen. Although each cell of the proximal tubule contains a large spherical nucleus, not all cells in a given section of a tubule show a nuclear profile because of the large size of component cells.

The other major tubular component associated with the cortex is the **distal convoluted tubule**. It is shorter than the proximal convoluted tubule, therefore fewer profiles are seen in histologic preparations. The lumen of the distal convoluted tubule generally is wider than that of the proximal tubules, the cells are shorter and lighter staining, and nuclear profiles usually are seen in each cell. Cells of the distal tubule lack a brush (microvillus) border. With special staining methods, such as iron hematoxylin, a well-developed system of **basal striations** can be demonstrated in cells forming the distal convoluted tubule.

Return to the low-power objective and locate and examine several renal corpuscles for vascular poles as well as portions of the distal tubules located immediately adjacent to these structures. This region of the distal tubule (the pars maculata) may contain a section through the **macula densa**. Cells of the macula densa are taller and narrower than those in adjacent tubules and their **nuclei are crowded together at the apex** of the cells. Several renal corpuscles may have to be examined with the low power objective before a macula densa can be located. Look for four to eight dense-staining nuclei crowded together and bordering the lumen of the lighter-staining distal tubule. Next, examine the afferent and efferent arterioles of the vascular pole. The macula densa is related to (lies next to) a modified region of the afferent arteriole that may contain **juxtaglomerular (JG) cells**. JG cells are highly modified smooth muscle cells in the wall of the afferent arteriole located where it enters the renal corpuscle. The JG cells are located in the tunica media, are light staining, cuboidal in shape and contain a number of secretory granules. Due to the plane of section, more often than not, the macula densa and JG cells will not be found together but appear to occur as independent entities. It should be remembered that all of the structures considered thus far; renal corpuscles, proximal convoluted tubules, distal convoluted tubules, macula densa and JG cells, occur **ONLY in the cortex**.

Make a composite sketch that illustrates all the histologic features normally associated with a renal corpuscle and the relationships of several of these structures.

Compare the sketches made of the glomerulus with photographs taken with a scanning electron microscope that illustrate the glomerular epithelium, glomerular endothelium and the shared basement membrane.

Next examine the **medulla** of the kidney with the low-power objective and observe that unlike the tubules of the cortex, those forming the medulla lie parallel to one another. Identify the three tubules normally associated with the medulla: thin segments, thick segments (first part of the distal tubule) and medullary collecting tubules. The **medullary**

collecting tubules are the most obvious and are lined by a light-staining simple columnar epithelium. They are further characterized by distinct cell boundaries between individual cells. As the medullary collecting ducts pass through the medulla toward the renal papilla they converge to form larger, straight collecting ducts called **papillary ducts**. The lining epithelium of these ducts transitions from tall simple columnar to stratified columnar to transitional epithelium at the tip of the renal papillae where the epithelium of the ducts becomes continuous with that covering the external surface of the papillae. Note that a few collecting tubules extend (within medullary rays) into the cortex. These exhibit the same morphologic features as those observed in the medulla. Return to the medulla and identify numerous tubules lined by a light-gray staining cuboidal epithelium whose nuclei touch both the basal and apical cell membranes. Intercellular boundaries are indistinct. These tubules form the first portion of the **distal tubule** (pars recta) and sometimes are referred to as the thick ascending limb of the loop of Henle. Examine the medulla carefully with the high-power objective for **thin segments** (of the loop of Henle). These can be found in the interstitial connective tissue hidden between the other two tubules. They exhibit a much smaller diameter ($\sim$20 μm) and are lined by a **thin simple squamous epithelium** that bounds an irregularly shaped lumen. Nuclei of the lining epithelial cells are centrally placed and cause this area of the cell to bulge into the lumen of the tubule.

Examine the medulla and cortex for its **vascular supply**. Re-examine the cortex for renal corpuscles and identify the associated afferent and efferent arterioles. Examine several until an **afferent arteriole** is located that can be traced to elongated arterioles running perpendicular to the outer surface of the cortex. These vessels are **interlobular arteries**. Next examine the corticomedullary junction for transverse sections of arteries and veins of much larger caliber. These vessels are **arcuate vessels**. With the high-power objective examine the medulla for thin-walled vessels, about the size of thin segments, that occur in groups and usually contain numerous erythrocytes. These vessels are the **vasa recta**.

Make a sketch of the observations made in the renal medulla. Construct an additional composite sketch illustrating the vasculature associated with both the cortex and medulla of the kidney.

Table 16. Key histologic features of structures found in the kidney.			
Structure	**Primary location**	**Features of epithelium**	**Other features**
Proximal convoluted tubule	Cortex	Large granular, dark-staining cells; brush border; not all cells show a nuclear profile	Stellate or irregular lumen
Distal convoluted tubule	Cortex	Light-staining columnar cells that lack a brush-border; each cell shows a nuclear profile	Smooth luminal surface, large and circular in outline
Renal corpuscles (Bowman s capsule, glomerulus)	Cortex	Glomerular epithelium exhibits light-staining nuclei; glomerular endothelium exhibits dark-staining nuclei	Vascular and urinary poles, thick basement membrane
Thin segment (loop of Henle)	Medulla	Light-staining tubule lined by simple squamous epithelium	Narrow lumen
Thick segment (loop of Henle)	Medulla	Light-staining tubule lined by simple cuboidal epithelium	Wide, round lumen
Collecting tubule	Medulla	Light-staining columnar cells, distinct cell boundaries	Large, round lumen

Extrarenal passages

The extrarenal passages consist of the minor and major calyces, the renal pelvis, ureters, urinary bladder and urethra.

With the exception of the urethra, all consist of a mucosa, muscularis and adventitia. These three layers are thinnest in the minor calyces and increase in depth distally reaching their greatest depth in the urinary bladder. Beginning with the lumen examine the mucosa of each of these structures. The **mucosa** consists of a **transitional epithelium** lying on a **lamina propria**, the connective tissue of which blends with that enveloping the bundles of **smooth muscle** of the **muscularis**. The lamina propria consists of a compact layer of fibroelastic tissue. The muscularis consists of two layers of smooth muscle, an inner longitudinal layer and an outer circular layer, in the minor and major calyces, renal pelvis and proximal ureters. In the lower one-third of the ureter an outer longitudinal layer appears in the muscularis. Like the distal ureter, the muscularis of the urinary bladder consists of inner longitudinal, middle circular, and outer longitudinal layers of smooth muscle. The

middle layer is the most prominent. The **adventitia**, a coat of fibroelastic connective tissue, surrounds the muscularis and functions to attach the extrarenal passages to surrounding structures. The adventitia of the ureters and urinary bladder is an excellent place to find small blood vessels, nerves and small ganglia for examination and review.

Sketch a transverse section through the ureter. Determine the region from which the sample of ureter was taken.

The **urethra of the male** is subdivided into three regions dependent on its position : prostatic urethra, membranous urethra and penile urethra. The **prostatic urethra** is lined by transitional epithelium and lies within the substance of the prostate (an accessory sex gland). The **membranous urethra** is short and extends from the apex of the prostate to the root of the penis. In doing so it passes through the skeletal muscle of the urogenital diaphragm. It is lined by either stratified or pseudostratified columnar epithelium. The **penile urethra** runs longitudinally through the erectile tissue of the corpus spongiosum and is lined by a pseudostratified columnar epithelium.

Patches of non-keratinized stratified squamous epithelium often occur especially near its distal end. The lamina propria is a highly vascular, loose collagenous connective tissue rich in elastic fibers. The epithelial lining of the urethra often contains small evaginations which are continuous with **intraepithelial nests (glands of Littr)** of clear-mucous-secreting cells. The mucosa is bounded by poorly defined inner longitudinal and outer circular layers of smooth muscle that separate it from adjacent erectile tissue.

The **female urethra** is lined by stratified squamous epithelium, although patches of stratified or pseudostratified columnar may be found. Glands of Littr also are present. The lamina propria is a vascular fibroelastic connective tissue that contains numerous venous sinuses. A poorly defined muscularis, consisting inner longitudinal and outer circular bundles of smooth muscle, also occurs. The female urethra may be surrounded by skeletal muscle of the urogenital diaphragm.

Table 17. Key histologic features of the extrarenal passages.		
Region	**Epithelium**	**Supporting wall**
Ureter (proximal two-thirds)	Transitional (4-5 cell layers)	Inner longitudinal and outer circular layers of smooth muscle
Ureter (distal one-third)	Transitional (4-5 cell layers)	Inner longitudinal, middle circular and outer longitudinal layers of smooth muscle
Urinary bladder	Transitional (8 or more cell layers)	Inner longitudinal, middle circular and outer longitudinal layers of smooth muscle
Male urethra Pars prostatica	Transitional	Prostate
Pars membranacea	Stratified/pseudostratified stratified columnar	Skeletal muscle of sphincter urethrae
Pars cavernosa	Stratified and/or pseudostratified columnar; patches of wet stratified squamous in fossa navicularis	Erectile tissue of corpus cavernosum urethrae
Female urethrae	Stratified columnar; wet stratified squamous epithelium	Inner longitudinal and outer circular layer of smooth muscle

The male reproductive system consists of the testes, an excurrent duct system, accessory sex glands and external genitalia.

Learning objectives for the male reproductive system:

1. Be able to identify and describe the general histologic architecture of the testis.
2. Be able to identify and describe the cell types comprising the germinal epithelium of seminiferous tubules.
3. Be able to identify and describe the interstitial tissue and Leydig cells.
4. Be able to identify and describe the histologic structure of the different regions constituting the excurrent duct system that links the testis to the urethra.
5. Be able to identify and describe the histologic structure of the male accessory sex glands.

Testes

The testes are bounded by a thick capsule called the **tunica albuginea**, which consists of dense fibroelastic connective tissue with scattered smooth muscle cells. The external surface of the tunica albuginea may be covered by a simple squamous epithelium (mesothelium), the visceral layer of **tunica vaginalis**. Adjacent to the inner region of the tunica albuginea lies the **tunica vasculosa**, a region of loose connective tissue that contains numerous small blood vessels. Continue to examine the remainder of the testis under low power and observe that it consists of numerous seminiferous tubules separated by a delicate **interstitial tissue** rich in small blood and lymphatic vessels. Select and examine several regions of the interstitial tissue at increased magnification. Observe that it contains fibroblasts, macrophages, mast cells and large polyhedral cells 15 to 20 μm in diameter called **interstitial cells (of Leydig)**. These may occur singly, or more commonly in groups, and make up the endocrine portion of the testis secreting the male hormone, testosterone. Human interstitial cells are characterized by large cytoplasmic crystals called the **crystals of Reinke**. Although highly variable in size and shape, they are readily seen as slightly darker structures in the light-staining cytoplasm of the interstitial cell. Return to low power and examine the section of testis for the **mediastinum testis**. The mediastinum represents a thickening of the tunica albuginea that projects into the testis from the posterior region. Numerous, thin connective tissue partitions, called **septula testis**, extend from the mediastinum which subdivide the testis into pyramidal-shaped compartments called **lobuli testis**.

Make a sketch illustrating these features.

Return to a **seminiferous tubule** and examine it at increased magnification. Beginning at the periphery of the tubule note the nature of the thin collagen fibers and flattened cells of the **peritubular tissue** bounding the seminiferous tubule.

The **germinal epithelium** of the seminiferous tubules is unique among epithelia in that it consists of a fixed population of supporting cells, called Sertoli cells, and a proliferating population of differentiating spermatogenic cells.

The **Sertoli cell** is tall and spans the height of the germinal epithelium, reaching from the basement membrane to the luminal surface. This cell type has an elaborate shape and envelopes adjacent differentiating spermatogenic cells. The extent of the cytoplasmic boundaries **cannot be seen** with the light microscope. The Sertoli cell does, however, exhibit a prominent, characteristic nucleus that **is key** to its identification. The nucleus is large, elongate, irregular in shape and is distinguished by a **large, prominent nucleolus**.

Spermatogenic cells extend from the basement membrane to the luminal surface of the germinal epithelium and are subdivided into several categories: spermatogonia, primary spermatocytes, secondary spermatocytes and spermatids. **Spermatogonia** lie on the basement membrane between the bases of adjacent Sertoli cells, are round or elliptical in shape, and measure 10 to 20 μm in diameter. Two types of spermatogonia can be differentiated by the characteristics of their nuclei. **Type A** spermatogonia have spherical or elliptical nuclei with a fine chromatin pattern and one or two nucleoli located near the nuclear envelope. Many nuclei of this cell type also exhibit a **clear nuclear vacuole**. Nuclei of **type B** spermatogonia are spherical, light staining and contain variable-sized clumps of chromatin, most of which are arranged along the nuclear envelope. A single, centrally placed nucleolus may be observed on occasion. **Primary spermatocytes** usually are found in the basal half of the germinal epithelium and are the largest spherical cells observed. All exist in some state of meiosis and threadlike chromosomes are a characteristic observation. In contrast to primary spermatocytes, which are numerous, **secondary spermatocytes** are a rare observation due to their rapid division into spermatids.

When seen, secondary spermatocytes appear similar to but are about half the size of the primary spermatocytes and are located nearer the lumen of the seminiferous tubule. Numerous spermatids at different stages of maturation are found scattered within the germinal epithelium. **Early spermatids** are about one half the size of secondary spermatocytes and exhibit round nuclei one surface of which may be associated with a forming acrosome. Early spermatids may be found on occasion near the center of the germinal epithelium. **Late spermatids** exhibit well-defined head and tail regions and appear very similar to spermatozoa observed in the lumen of the seminiferous tubules following their release by Sertoli cells. Late spermatids often border the lumen of the seminiferous tubule.

Sketch a transverse section through a seminiferous tubule illustrating the position of Sertoli cell nuclei and their relationship to the various spermatogenic cells within the germinal epithelium.

Excurrent duct system

Excurrent ducts link the testes to the urethra and consist of the tubuli recti (straight tubules), rete testis, ductus efferentes, ductus epididymidis, ductus deferens and the ejaculatory ducts.

Near the apex of each testicular lobule, the seminiferous tubules lack spermatogenic cells and consist only of a simple columnar lining epithelium of Sertoli cells. These short, straight tubules are referred to as **tubuli recti**. The lumina of the tubuli recti are continuous with a system of anastomosing channels, the **rete testis**, found in the mediastinum. The channels of the rete testis are surrounded by a dense bed of vascular connective tissue and are lined by a **dark-staining, simple cuboidal epithelium**. The channels of the rete testis merge to form 10 to 15 ductuli efferentes, which in turn unite to form a single ductus epididymidis. The **efferent ductules** form the initial portion (head) of the epididymis. The lumen of the efferent ductule exhibits a characteristic irregular contour due to the presence of alternating groups of **tall** and **short columnar cells**. Both **ciliated and nonciliated cells are present**. The efferent ductule is bounded by a thin layer of **circularly arranged smooth muscle** that thickens toward the ductus epididymidis. A scant connective tissue lamina propria separates the lining epithelium from the surrounding smooth muscle cells.

Examine a section of **epididymis** at low power and note that it consists of numerous tubular profiles separated by a delicate connective tissue. It is important to realize that these profiles are of a single **ductus epididymidis**, that if uncoiled, measures 5 - 7 m in length. The epithelial lining is **pseudostratified columnar** and consists of basal and principal cells. Scan the entire epididymis and determine if the epithelial lining is of the same height in all tubular profiles examined. **Principal cells** are the most numerous and very tall (80 μm) in the proximal region of the ductus epididymidis but gradually decrease in height to measure only 40 μm near its junction with the vas deferens. Long, branched microvilli, called **stereocilia**, extend from the apical surfaces of the principal cells. **Basal cells** are small, round cells that lie on the basement membrane interposed between the bases of principal cells. A thin layer of circularly arranged **smooth muscle** surrounds a thin lamina propria. The muscle layer thickens near the ductus deferens and becomes organized into three layers. Note that spermatozoa are often found clustered in the lumen of the ductus epididymidis.

The **ductus deferens** is characterized by a thick wall consisting of a mucosa, a muscularis and an adventitia. The **mucosa** is in the form of longitudinal folds that extend into a small lumen and are covered by a **pseudostratified columnar epithelium**. Note that it is similar in appearance to that of the ductus epididymidis. The underlying lamina propria is compact and contains numerous elastic fibers. The **muscularis** forms the majority of the wall and consists of **three layers of smooth muscle** arranged longitudinally in the outer and inner layers and circularly in the middle layer. Recall that for its size the ductus deferens is considered the most muscular tube in the body. The muscularis is surrounded by an **adventitia** of loose connective tissue. In the **ampulla** of the ductus deferens (the distal-most region of the ductus deferens) the lumen expands and the mucosa is highly folded, creating a labyrinth of pocket like recesses. The histologic features of the wall remain the same as elsewhere in the ductus deferens. The muscle wall, however, is thinner.

A short, narrow region of the ductus deferens extends beyond the ampulla and unites with the duct of the seminal vesicle forming a short tube about 1 cm in length called the **ejaculatory duct**. It is lined by a pseudostratified or stratified columnar epithelium with the remainder of the wall consisting only of dense collagenous connective tissue.

Sketch and compare a transverse section through each of the following excurrent tubules detailing the lining epithelium and the constituents forming the limiting wall: rete testis, ductus efferentes, ductus epididymidis and ductus deferens.

Table 18. Key histologic features of the male reproductive system.

Region	Epithelial lining	Support	Muscle
Seminiferous tubule	Germinal epithelium containing spermatogenic cells (spermatogonia, primary and secondary spermatocytes, spermatids) and Sertoli cells	Peritubular connective tissue; collagen fibers and myoid cells. Leydig cells in adjacent interstitial tissue between seminiferous tubules	Absent
Tubuli recti	Simple columnar, consisting of Sertoli cells	Loose connective tissue	Absent
Rete testis	Simple cuboidal. Short microvilli, single cilium on each cell	Dense, vascular connective tissue	Absent
Ductuli efferentes	Lining has an irregular contour. Simple epithelium of tall, ciliated columnar and short ciliated or nonciliated cuboidal cells	Loose connective tissue between tubules	Thin, circular smooth muscle
Ductus epididymidis	Pseudostratified columnar: tall principal cells with stereocilia; short basal cells	Thin lamina propria	Primarily circular smooth muscle, three layers appear distally
Ductus deferens	Pseudostratified columnar, thrown into longitudinal folds; stereocilia	Dense lamina propria, collagen and elastic fibers; adventitia of loose connective tissue	Three layers: inner longitudinal, middle circular, outer longitudinal smooth muscle
Ampulla of ductus deferens	Pseudostratified columnar with stereocilia; complex folds form extensive pocket-like recesses	Lamina propria and adventitia less well defined	Thinner, less distinct layers of smooth muscle
Ejaculatory duct	Pseudostratified or stratified columnar; may form pockets but less prominent than in ampulla	Dense collagenous connective tissue with many elastic fibers	Absent

Accessory sex glands

Male accessory sex glands include the seminal vesicles, prostate and bulbourethral glands.

Seminal vesicles

The seminal vesicles are elongated, sac-like structures that lie posterior to the prostate. The **mucosa** of the seminal vesicle is characterized by being organized into a system of complex primary, secondary and tertiary folds that subdivide the lumen into many small, irregularly shaped compartments. The epithelial lining is mainly pseudostratified columnar although regions of simple columnar epithelium also occur. The epithelium rests on a thin **lamina propria** rich in elastic fibers bounded by a **coat of smooth muscle** organized into inner circular and outer longitudinal layers. A layer of loose connective tissue lies on the external surface on the muscle wall.

Make a sketch of a region from the seminal vesicle illustrating these features.

Prostate

The prostate is a **composite gland**, made up of 30 to 50 small, **compound tubuloalveolar glands**. These small glands form strata around the urethra and are organized into periurethral mucosal glands, submucosal glands and the principal prostatic glands, which make up the bulk of the prostate and lie at the periphery. The light-staining **glandular epithelium varies** from gland to gland and even in a single alveolus. It varies from simple or pseudostratified columnar but may be low cuboidal or squamous in some regions. The lumina of the secretory units may contain **prostatic concretions**, solid spherical bodies of condensed secretory material. Individual glands are separated by a **fibromuscular stroma** rich in smooth muscle cells and is **characteristic** of the prostate. The prostate is contained within a vascular, fibroelastic capsule that contains an abundance of smooth muscle along its interior. Broad septa extend from the capsule into the prostate and blend with the fibromuscular stroma.

Make a detailed sketch of a region of the prostate illustrating in particular the fibromuscular stroma and prostatic concretions.

Bulbourethral glands

Bulbourethral glands are **compound tubuloalveolar glands** located in skeletal muscle of the urogenital diaphragm. The glandular epithelium ranges from **simple cuboidal** to **simple columnar** depending of the functional state of these glands and whether or not the alveoli are distended by contained secretory product. In routine preparations active cells are light staining and filled with unstained mucin granules that compress the nucleus to the base of the cell. Each gland is limited by a connective tissue capsule from which septa extend dividing the glands into lobules. The capsule and septa may contain smooth and skeletal muscle cells interspersed within the connective tissue elements.

Penis

The penile urethra lies within a cylinder of erectile tissue, the **corpus spongiosum (corpus cavernosum urethrae)** positioned ventral to a pair of similar erectile bodies called the **corpora cavernosa penis**. These three structures make up the bulk of the penis. The two corpora cavernosa penis are united by a common dense connective tissue septum called the **pectiniform septum**. A thick, dense collagenous sheath, the tunica albuginea, limits each of the three corpora. Observe that the three corpora are bound together by subcutaneous connective tissue rich in smooth muscle cells. **Trabeculae** consisting of collagenous fibers, elastic fibers and smooth muscle cells extend from the tunica albuginea and divide the interior of the corpora cavernosa into numerous **cavernous spaces**, the larger of which are located near the center of the erectile body. The cavernous spaces are endothelial-lined vascular spaces continuous with the arteries that supply them and with veins draining them. Identify the highly convoluted **helicine arteries** (arterioles) that lie within the trabeculae of the cavernous tissue. These vessels are characterized by long, ridgelike thickenings of the intima that project into and partially occlude the lumina. The **intimal ridges** are most frequent where the helicine arteries branch and consist of a core of loose connective tissue that contains an abundance of smooth muscle cells underlying the endothelium. Veins are most commonly found along the interior of the tunica albuginea. A fold of hairless skin called the prepuce (foreskin) covers the distal enlargement of the corpus spongiosum, the glans penis. The keratinized stratified squamous epithelium covering the glans contains numerous free nerve endings and is associated with Meissner's corpuscles. Vater-Pacini corpuscles are present in the deeper layers of the dermis.

Table 19. Key histologic features of accessory structures associated with the male reproductive system.

Region	Epithelial lining	Support	Muscle
Prostate	Variable; usually simple columnar or pseudostratified columnar. Low cuboidal or squamous cells may occur. Prostatic concretions occur in lumen of glands	Vascular connective tissue with dense network of elastic fibers	Smooth muscle cells in connective tissue surrounding individual glandular units (fibromuscular stroma)
Seminal vesicles	Honeycombed appearance; pseudostratified columnar with regions of simple columnar	Thin lamina propria with many elastic fibers; external layer of loose connective tissue rich in elastic fibers	Inner circular and outer longitudinal layers of smooth muscle form the limiting wall
Bulbourethral glands	Variable; simple cuboidal to simple columnar; flattened in distended alveoli; ducts lined by simple columnar, pseudostratified near urethra	Fibroelastic connective tissue around each glandular structure	Smooth and skeletal muscle fibers in interstitial tissue between glandular elements
Corpus cavernosa penis	Endothelium of vascular spaces	Fibroelastic connective tissue	Smooth muscle cells in trabeculae between cavernous spaces
Corpus cavernosa urethrae	Penile urethrae lined by either stratified or pseudostratified columnar, or wet stratified squamous; cavernous spaces lined by endothelium	Fibroelastic connective tissue rich in elastic fibers	Smooth muscle cells more abundant in trabeculae between cavernous spaces

The female reproductive tract consists of the ovaries, oviducts, uterus, vagina and external genitalia. The mammary glands are important accessory organs of the female reproductive system.

Learning objectives for the female reproductive system:

1. Be able to recognize and describe the histologic structure of the ovary.

2. Be able to recognize and describe the morphologic differences that occur between ovarian follicles at different stages of maturation through ovulation.

3. Be able to recognize and describe follicles that have undergone atresia.

4. Be able to recognize and describe a corpus luteum and understand its transformation (luteinization) from a ruptured mature follicle.

5. Be able to recognize and describe the structural organization of the oviduct (Fallopian tube) and the changes that occur along its length.

6. Be able to recognize and describe the structural organization of the uterine wall.

7. Be able to recognize and describe the structural organization of the endometrium and the histologic changes that occur during the three primary phases of the uterine cycle (proliferative, secretory and menstrual phases).

8. Be able to recognize and describe the histologic organization of the cervix and vaginal wall as well as the junction between these structures.

9. Be able to recognize and describe the histologic organization of the placenta in early and late pregnancy.

10. Be able recognize and describe the major histologic changes that occur in the female breast as a result of pregnancy and during lactation.

Ovaries

Examine the ovary with the low-power objective and observe that it consists of a peripheral darker-staining **cortex** that contains **ovarian follicles** whose size varies with their stage of development. Note that the external surface of the ovary is covered by a **surface epithelium** of simple cuboidal cells. The connective tissue underlying the surface epithelium is less cellular, more compact and forms a dense fibrous layer, referred to as the **tunica albuginea**. The central, lighter-staining region of the ovary, the **medulla**, consists of a loose connective tissue that houses numerous blood vessels, lymphatics and nerves. Note that the follicles are located only in the cortex, deep to the tunica albuginea, and that each consists of a central

ovum surrounded by one or more layers of epithelial cells. Examine the different categories of follicles at increased magnification. **Primordial** or **unilaminar follicles** lie just beneath the tunica albuginea and consist of a **central ovum** surrounded by a **single layer of flattened follicular cells**. In contrast, **primary follicles** are identified by follicular cells, which become cuboidal or columnar in shape and may form one to several layers of cells. The follicular cells are now termed **granulosa cells** and the stratified layer they form is referred to as the **stratum granulosum**. A structureless refractile membrane, the **zona pellucida**, lies between the central ovum and the adjacent follicular cells. In larger-growing primary follicles the adjacent ovarian stroma becomes organized into a sheath, the **theca folliculi**. Examine this thin fibrous layer carefully and observe that it can be subdivided into an inner, slightly more cellular layer, called the **theca interna** and an outer fibrous layer, the **theca externa**. Note that cells of the theca interna are plumper and may contain small lipid droplets as well as the presence of **numerous capillaries** associated with this layer. The boundary between these two layers is indistinct and the theca externa merges with the surrounding stroma. Observe that as the follicles increase in size they are located deeper in the cortex. As the stratum granulosum becomes eight to ten cell layers thick, fluid-filled spaces appear between granulosa cells with continued growth of the follicle. As these spaces increase in size they merge to form a single cavity called the **follicular antrum**. Large follicles that exhibit such a cavity are termed **antral** or **secondary follicles**. Secondary follicles continue to increase in size and the follicular antrum expands. Eventually the ovum becomes eccentrically placed in the follicle, surrounded by a mass of granulosa cells called the **cumulus oophorus**, which remains continuous with those lining the antral cavity. Granulosa cells that immediately surround the oocyte form the **corona radiata** and are separated from it by a well-developed **zona pellucida**. Examine the changes that have occurred in the theca folliculi. The foregoing features characterize the **mature (Graafian) follicle**.

Draw a series of labeled sketches illustrating the progressive changes that occur during follicular development beginning with a primordial follicle and ending with a mature follicle.

It should be realized that the majority of follicles undergo a degenerative process called **atresia**, which may occur at any stage in the development of a follicle. Examine several follicles for signs of atresia.

During atresia of a primary follicle, the ovum shrinks and shows signs of cytolysis, as do the surrounding granulosa cells. Similar changes occur in larger follicles, but in this instance the zona pellucida may persist for some time after dissolution of the oocyte and follicular cells. Macrophages commonly are seen invading atretic follicles and contain degenerative material, including fragments of the zona pellucida. During atresia, cells of the theca interna persist longer than those of the stratum granulosum but also show degenerative changes. Thecal cells increase in size, lipid droplets accumulate in their cytoplasm and the cells assume an epithelioid character. Groups of thecal cells can become separated by connective tissue fibers and capillaries. The basement membrane that lies between the stratum granulosum and the theca interna frequently becomes thicker and forms a hyalinized, corrugated layer called the **glassy membrane**. The glassy membrane is characteristic of growing follicles that have undergone atresia and aids in distinguishing a large atretic follicle from the corpus luteum.

Following ovulation, the walls of the mature follicle collapse, are thrown into folds and may surround a central blood clot. The ruptured follicle is transformed into a structure known as a corpus luteum by a process called luteinization. The **corpus luteum** is a large structure, about the size of a fingernail, and readily seen by direct observation of the section prior to putting it under the microscope. Granulosa cells increase greatly in size, become polyhedral in shape, and are transformed into pale-staining **granulosa lutein cells**. Cells of the theca interna also enlarge and become epithelioid in nature forming **theca lutein cells**. They are smaller in size than the granulosa lutein cells. Theca lutein cells are organized peripherally, and are abundant in the recesses between the folds of granulosa lutein cells. Observe that capillaries from the theca interna invade the lutein tissue to form a complex, delicate vascular network in the corpus luteum. Connective tissue from the theca interna also penetrates the mass of lutein cells and forms a delicate network about them. If pregnancy does not occur the corpus luteum undergoes involution in about 14 days. In this case the lutein cells decrease in size, accumulate lipid droplets and degenerate. Hyaline material accumulates between lutein cells, connective tissue cells become dense and pyknotic and the corpus luteum is replaced by a white scar of dense connective tissue called a **corpus albicans**.

Sketch a region of the corpus luteum and compare and contrast the position and structure of granulosa and theca lutein cells.

Table 20. Key histologic features of ovarian structures.

Structure	Ovum	Cells of wall	Other
Primordial follicle	Dominates follicle; nucleus large, central and vesicular; prominent nucleolus	Unilaminar layer of flattened follicular cells	
Primary follicle	Large with central vesicular nucleus; zona pellucida may be visible	One or more layers of granulosa cells; cuboidal in shape	Surrounding stoma organized into theca interna and externa
Secondary follicle	Large vesicular nucleus; zona pellucida prominent	Stratum granulosum 8 to 12 cell layers thick; large spaces between cells; formation of antrum	Well defined theca interna and externa
Mature follicle	Ovum eccentric in large follicle located near surface of ovary	Granulosa cells organized into cumulus oophorus and corona radiata; very large antrum	Well defined theca interna and externa; cells of theca interna plump
Atretic follicle	May or may not be present; show signs of degeneration	Show degenerative changes; macrophages usually present; connective tissue infiltration	Cells of theca interna show degenerative changes; appearance of glassy membrane
Corpus luteum	Absent	Prominent granulosa lutein cells; smaller theca lutein cells	Vascularization of the corpus luteum
Corpus albicans	Absent	Thin, dark staining nuclei of fibroblasts	Large bundles of thin collagen fibers; hyaline material

Oviducts

The oviducts (uterine tubes) are a pair of muscular tubes that link the ovaries to the uterus. The oviduct is divided into four regions: the **infundibulum**, a funnel-shaped region with its margin drawn out into numerous tapering processes called fimbria; the **ampulla**, a tortuous, thin-walled segment that makes up about half the length of the oviduct; the **isthmus**, a narrow region that makes up the medial one-third; and the **intramural (interstitial) region**, located in the uterine wall. The wall of the oviduct consists of an internal mucosa, an intermediate muscularis and an external serosa.

The **mucosa** of the oviduct is in the form of longitudinal folds called **plicae**. In the ampulla note that the plicae have secondary and tertiary folds and create a complex labyrinth of epithelial-lined spaces. In the isthmus, plicae are shorter with less branching and in the intramural region appear only as low ridges.

The entire oviduct is lined by a **ciliated simple columnar epithelium** that rests on delicate lamina propria rich in fibroblasts. The epithelium decreases in height distally in the oviduct and consists of both **ciliated** and **non-ciliated** cells. Non-ciliated cells are narrow and peg-shaped, and their apical cytoplasm often bulges into the lumen. The narrow nuclei often appear more deeply stained and are positioned nearer the lumen than those of ciliated cells. As a result, these cells are often referred to as **"peg"** cells. The mucosa rests directly on the **muscularis**, which consists of **inner circular** and **outer longitudinal** layers of smooth muscle. Externally, the oviduct is covered by a **serosa**.

Make a labeled sketch of the oviduct. Determine the region of the oviduct examined.

Uterus

The uterus, like the oviduct, consists of different regions. The majority of the uterus consists of the **body**, the upper expanded portion. The dome-shaped region of the body above the entrance points of the oviducts is referred to as the **fundus**. Distally, the uterus narrows, becomes cylindrical in shape and partially protrudes into the vagina and forms the **cervix**. The wall of the uterus is made up of three basic layers: a mucosa or *endometrium*, a middle muscle layer or *myometrium*, and a serosa or *perimetrium*.

The **endometrium** is a complex mucous membrane, the structure of which undergoes cyclic changes. It is lined by a **simple columnar epithelium** that consists of ciliated cells and non-ciliated secretory cells. **Uterine glands** extend from this surface deep into the underlying stroma of the endometrium. Most are simple tubular glands, but some may branch near the myometrium. There are fewer ciliated cells in the epithelium forming these glands than observed in the lining epithelium. The **endometrial stroma** resembles mesenchymal tissue and consists of loosely arranged stellate cells with large, round or ovoid nuclei. These cells are enveloped by fine connective tissue fibers. Lymphocytes, granular leukocytes and macrophages are often found scattered within the stroma. The endometrium can be subdivided into two layers: a stratum basale (basal layer) and a stratum functionale (functional layer). The **stratum basale** is narrower, more cellular, more fibrous and lies immediately adjacent to the myometrium. Note that when viewed at low power it is darker staining when compared to the functionalis. Small areas of stratum basale may be encountered extending into the myometrium, between bundles of smooth muscle cells. The **stratum functionalis** is much thicker and extends from the lumen of the uterus to the stratum basale. With the high-power objective examine the endometrial stroma of the functionalis for **spiral arteries**. These can be found by looking for groups of transverse profiles of arterioles closely packed together which represent a single, highly coiled arteriole lying in the stroma between uterine glands.

Observe that the majority of the uterine wall consists of **myometrium**. This smooth muscle wall measures 15 - 20 mm in depth and is formed by several poorly defined layers united by smooth muscle cells that intermingle. Generally, inner, middle and outer layers can be distinguished.

The **perimetrium** corresponds to the serosal layer covering the uterus.

Make a detailed sketch of the endometrium.

Questions: Can the stage of the cycle be determined from the section examined? How do the glands differ? How does the stroma differ?

Cervix

A section through the wall of the **cervix** differs considerably from one taken through the body of the uterus. Note that little smooth muscle is present in the **cervical wall** and that it **consists** mainly **of dense connective tissue**. A mucosa or endocervix lines the lumen of the cervical canal, which is in the form of complex branching folds. The epithelial lining consists primarily of **tall, light-staining, mucus-secreting columnar cells**. Large, branching **cervical glands** are present in the mucosa that are formed by mucus-secreting cells similar to those of the lining epithelium. On occasion some glands become occluded and filled with secretion, forming Nabothian cysts. The region of the cervix that extends into the vaginal canal is covered by a **nonkeratinized stratified squamous epithelium** on its external surface.

*Find, examine and sketch the **abrupt transition** of the simple columnar epithelium within the cervical canal to the non-keratinized stratified squamous epithelium covering the exterior surface of the cervix.*

Vagina

The wall of the **vagina** also consists of a mucosa, a muscularis and an adventitia. The **mucosa** consists of a **nonkeratinized stratified squamous epithelium** overlying a vascular **lamina propria** that consists of a fairly dense connective tissue which becomes more loosely arranged near the muscularis. Be aware that the vagina lacks glands. The **muscularis** consists of bundles of smooth muscle that are arranged into inner circular and outer longitudinal layers. The **adventitia** is a thin outer layer of connective tissue with abundant elastic fibers.

Table 21. Histologic features characteristic of the tubular portion of the female reproductive tract.			
Region	**Epithelial lining**	**Support**	**Organization of musculature in limiting wall**
Oviduct	Simple columnar; ciliated and nonciliated (peg) cells	Lamina propria cellular, thin collagen and reticular fibers	Well-defined inner circular layer of smooth muscle; outer layer of scattered longitudinal smooth muscle cells
Uterus	Simple columnar with groups of ciliated cells; extends into lamina propria to form tubular (uterine) glands	Lamina propria=endometrial stroma, similar to mesenchyme; richly cellular, fine reticular fibers, few collagen fibers. *Note*. The oviduct and uterus are the only hollow organs with this type of lamina propria	Myometrium; thick coat of smooth muscle with 3 intermingling layers
Cervix	1. Tall columnar mucus secreting cells lining endocervix 2. Vaginal part covered by non-keratinized stratified squamous	Dense collagenous and elastic connective tissue	Smooth muscle much reduced in amount, lacking in vaginal part
Vagina	Nonkeratinized stratified squamous	Vascular lamina propria of collagenous connective tissue. Dense elastic network below epithelial layer	Inner circular smooth muscle layer, outer longitudinal smooth muscle layer

Placenta

Examine an early placenta (prior to the 10th week of pregnancy) and concentrate primarily on finding and examining placental villi. Villi will appear as numerous, small irregular shaped structures making up the majority of the field. They consist of a delicate connective tissue core that contains small blood vessels (capillaries) and are covered by an epithelium that exhibits of two distinct cellular layers. The inner layer lies on a basement membrane and consists of large, discrete pale-staining cells, which form the **cytotrophoblast**. The outer covering layer, the **syncytial trophoblast**, is a darker-staining cellular layer of variable thickness in which prominent, small dense nuclei are present. In contrast to cells of the cytotrophoblast, intercellular boundaries cannot be distinguished in this layer. Re-examine the cores of several villi. Are nucleated erythrocytes present in the capillaries? Are large cells with large spherical nuclei present in the cores? Do they contain phagocytosed material? Recall that individual villi lie in lacunae through which maternal blood circulates. Are mature maternal erythrocytes present between and around the placental villi?

Examine and compare a region of a near-term placenta with a region from the early placenta. Observe that cells of the cytotrophoblast layer have disappeared and that the syncytial trophoblast thins out over the fetal capillaries at the periphery of villi to form a very thin layer. In other regions, it may become aggregated into protuberances referred to as syncytial knots. Masses of an eosinophilic, homogeneous substance called fibrinoid may be present on the external surface of some villi. Note that the erythrocytes within the capillaries of the villus core are now mature in appearance. At increased magnification examine the external surface of a placental villus and observe that only a very thin barrier exists (consisting of syncytial trophoblast, a basement membrane and an endothelial cell) that separates maternal from fetal blood. What is the functional significance of this region?

Make a detailed labeled sketch comparing sections through villi from early and term placentas.

Mammary gland

The mammary gland consists of 15 - 20 pyramidal-shaped lobes that radiate from a nipple. Each lobe represents an individual gland drained by its own ductal components. They are **compound tubuloalveolar glands** and are of cutaneous origin. In the **resting gland**, the major glandular constituents are the **ducts**, which are grouped together by surrounding connective tissue to form small **lobules**. Most of the smaller ducts are lined by a cuboidal epithelium which may become stratified in larger ducts nearer the nipple and in the lactiferous sinuses. The secretory units consist of clusters of small alveoli that closely surround the small ducts. The intralobular connective tissue around the ducts and alveoli is cellular and loosely arranged whereas that surrounding the larger ducts and lobes is variably dense and contains an abundance of adipose tissue. During the **first half of pregnancy**, the terminal portions of the ductal system grow rapidly, branch and begin to develop elongate alveoli. In **late pregnancy**, proliferation of glandular tissue decreases, the alveoli expand and there is some formation of secretory material by the lining epithelium. Fat and stromal connective tissue decrease in amount, and the remaining connective tissue becomes infiltrated with plasma cells, lymphocytes and granular leukocytes. A few days **following parturition** true milk secretion begins, but not all breast tissue functions at the same time. Note that in lactating tissue, some alveoli are distended by milk, the epithelial lining is flattened and the lumen distended. In other regions the alveoli are resting and lined by a simple columnar epithelium. Highly branched myoepithelial cells embrace alveoli and occur between the epithelium and the basement membrane.

Make three sketches comparing sections from a resting, pregnant and lactating mammary gland. Note in particular changes in the ductal system and secretory units.

Nipple

The nipple is covered by thin skin (**keratinized stratified squamous epithelium**) continuous with that covering the remainder of the breast. Unusually tall dermal papillae project into the epidermis of this region. The skin of the nipple is pigmented and contains numerous sebaceous glands but lacks hair follicles and sweat glands. Several **lactiferous ducts** traverse the nipple, each of which drains a lobe of the mammary gland via an expanded **lactiferous sinus** and empties onto the summit of the nipple. The latter generally are lined by stratified columnar but near the summit of the nipple, stratified squamous epithelium is often encountered. Note that the interior of the nipple consists of dense collagenous connective tissue, bundles of elastic fibers and a considerable amount of **smooth muscle**. Observe that the smooth muscle cells are arranged radially as well as circularly so that their contraction produces an erection of the nipple.

The **areola** is the pigmented, hairless region of skin encircling the base of the nipple. This region contains sebaceous, sweat and areolar glands. Note that the **areolar glands** are intermediate in structure between mammary glands and apocrine sweat glands.

Make a small sketch of the nipple region and any associated glands.

Classic endocrine glands lack ducts, and their secretions (hormones) enter the surrounding vasculature or lymphatic circulation. Their component cells present a relatively simple organization into either clumps, follicles, cords or plates enveloped by delicate vascular connective tissue.

Learning objectives for the classic endocrine glands:

1. Be able to recognize and describe the histologic details of the pineal gland.
2. Be able to recognize and describe the histologic details of the parathyroid glands.
3. Be able to recognize and describe the histologic details of the thyroid gland.
4. Be able to recognize and describe the histologic details of the adrenal glands. Be able to describe the vasculature associated with these glands.
5. Be able to recognize and describe the histologic details characteristic of each major subdivision of the pituitary gland (hypophysis).

Pineal gland

The pineal is covered by a thin capsule of connective tissue that is continuous with surrounding pial (meningeal) tissue. Observe that connective tissue septa extend from the capsule and subdivide the pineal into a series of poorly defined lobules. The parenchyma of this gland is organized into irregular cords and clumps consisting of two cell types, pinealocytes and glial cells. Examine a cord of parenchyma for **pinealocytes**. These cells are identified by their relatively large lobulated nuclei. With special staining techniques long cytoplasmic processes can be demonstrated that radiate from the cell body and form club-shaped endings near adjacent perivascular spaces or other pinealocytes. **Glial cells** form an interwoven network around and within the parenchymal cords and clumps of pinealocytes. They are fewer in number than pinealocytes and their nuclei are smaller and more deeply stained. Identify large, irregular concretions, the **corpora arenacea (brain sand)**, scattered in the capsule and substance of the pineal. These large acellular masses consist mainly of calcium carbonates and phosphates within an organic matrix.

Sketch a region of the pineal illustrating its histologic architecture.

Parathyroid glands

There are four or more of these small oval glands embedded within the capsule or substance of the thyroid gland. Each parathyroid gland is enveloped by a thin connective tissue capsule and is subdivided by delicate trabeculae that extend into its interior from the inner surface of the capsule. Observe that blood vessels, nerves and lymphatics course through the trabeculae to enter the parenchyma of the parathyroid. In elderly individuals, **fat cells** may be so abundant that they form 50% of the gland. The parenchyma itself consists of closely packed groups or branching cords of epithelial cells supported by a delicate connective tissue rich in reticular fibers. Note the rich capillary network intimately associated with the epithelial cords. The parenchyma of the parathyroid consists of two cell types: chief (principal) cells and oxyphil cells.

Chief (principal) cells are the more numerous and are identified by their centrally placed, round vesicular nuclei and light-staining cytoplasm. They are relatively small and measure 8 - 10 μm in diameter. **Oxyphil cells** form only a small population and may occur in groups or singly. Oxyphils are larger than chief cells and their cytoplasm stains intensely with eosin due to the large number of mitochondria in the cytoplasm. Note that their small nuclei stain intensely and often appear pyknotic.

Sketch and label a region of parathyroid containing both cell types.

Thyroid gland

The thyroid consists of two lateral lobes united by a narrow isthmus. The thyroid gland is enclosed by a thin connective tissue capsule. With the low-power objective observe that the parenchyma of the thyroid is organized into spherical structures called **follicles**. The follicles vary considerably in diameter and contain a darkly stained homogeneous material called **colloid**. Each follicle is invested and supported by a delicate reticular connective tissue that contains numerous capillaries. Examine the walls of several follicles using the high-power objective for these features. The follicular epithelium consists of a **single (simple) layer of principal (follicular) cells**. The latter may be squamous, cuboidal or columnar dependent on the functional status of the gland. Central nuclei are usually spherical in shape and contain one or more nucleoli. Close observation of the apical region may reveal **colloidal resorption droplets**, colloid taken up by the follicular cells. The thyroid also contains a smaller number of cells called **parafollicular, light or C cells**.

The latter occur either individually or in small groups (clusters) in the delicate connective tissue between follicles or scattered next to the follicular epithelium immediately adjacent to the basement membrane. Parafollicular cells never directly border the lumen of a follicle and are characterized by an abundant light staining cytoplasm and a central euchromatic nucleus.

Sketch and label the details of a thyroid follicle and of follicular and parafollicular cells.

Adrenal glands

Examine with low power and sketch an overview of this gland noting that it is surrounded by a capsule and that the gland is subdivided into two major regions, an outer dark-staining cortex and a central lighter-staining medulla. Examine the capsule at higher magnification and note that it is a relatively thick capsule of dense irregular connective tissue. Close observation of the capsule will reveal a rich plexus of blood vessels, particularly small arteries (arterioles), and numerous nerve fibers. Some arterioles and nerves enter the gland within trabeculae that extend into the cortex from the capsule and then leave the trabeculae to enter the parenchyma of the cortex. The parenchyma of the adrenal cortex is made up of continuous **cords of cells**, **separated by sinusoids** that extend from the capsule to the medulla.

Observe that the cortex is subdivided into three regions (zones) according to the organization of cells within the cords. Histologic changes from one zone to another are gradual. The **zona glomerulosa** forms a narrow layer just interior to the capsule and consists of columnar cells arranged into ovoid groups or arcades, component cells of which have centrally placed, spherical nuclei. The adjacent **zona fasciculata** forms the widest zone of the cortex and is comprised of long epithelial cords one to two cells thick. The cellular cords run parallel to one another and roughly perpendicular to the outer cortex and capsule. Well-developed sinusoids lie between and separate the epithelial cords of the zona fasciculata. Close examination of cells from this zone will demonstrate that they are larger than those of the zona glomerulosa and have a polyhedral shape. Nuclei are spherical and centrally placed within cells. Binucleate cells are not uncommon. Numerous lipid droplets characterize the cytoplasm of cells from this zone. In routine H&E preparations these appear as light-staining vacuoles (due to extraction of lipid as a result of processing) and because of this, have been termed spongiocytes. The innermost zone is called the **zona reticularis** and is formed by a network of irregular, anastomosing cords that are separated by sinusoids. Component cells resemble those of the zona

fasciculata but are smaller, the nuclei stain more intensely and the cytoplasm contains fewer lipid droplets.

Examine the **adrenal medulla** and observe that it is composed of large, round or polyhedral light-staining cells arranged into short cords or clumps. These are termed **chromaffin cells** because when treated with chromium salts in special staining procedures, numerous brown granules can be demonstrated within the cytoplasm of these cells. Examine the supporting framework of delicate connective tissue in the medulla and the numerous veins and nerve fibers present. Is a large central medullary vein present? **Sympathetic ganglion cells** may also be encountered either in small groups or singly. They can be identified as larger, lighter-staining cells with prominent euchromatic nuclei. Nucleoli are also a common observation in this cell type.

Re-examine the sinusoids and the entire blood supply associated with the adrenal gland. Trace the rich plexus of arterioles from the capsule to the parenchyma of the gland where they empty into a vast network of cortical sinusoids that separate cords of epithelial cells. Note that occasional arteries pass through the cortex to supply the medulla. Trace the sinusoids through all three zones of the cortex and observe that as they near the corticomedullary junction they begin to merge to form collecting veins. The collecting veins combine to form a single, large suprarenal vein that drains the entire adrenal gland.

Make a detailed, labeled sketch of the adrenal cortex and the associated medulla.

Pituitary (hypophysis)

The pituitary is a complex endocrine gland located at the base of the brain. It is attached to the hypothalamic region of the brain by a narrow stalk and has neural and vascular connections with the brain. The pituitary consists of two major components: an epithelial component called the **adenohypophysis** and a nervous component known as the **neurohypophysis**. The adenohypophysis is further **subdivided** into the **pars distalis (anterior lobe)** that lies anterior to a thin region characterized by cysts called the **pars intermedia**, and the **pars tuberalis** a continuation of epithelial cells from the pars distalis that extends to and around the neural stalk. The **neurohypophysis** also **consists** of three parts. A major bulbus part, the **pars nervosa**, which lies just posterior to the **pars intermedia** and is continuous with the **infundibular stalk**, and the **median eminence**. The entire pituitary is surrounded by a thick connective tissue capsule.

With low power, determine the plane section through the pituitary and determine which subcomponents are present in the section.

Make a sketch of those present noting their relationships to one another before examining each subcomponent at a higher magnification.

Pars distalis (anterior lobe)

The pars distalis consists of epithelial cells arranged in irregular cords and clumps. These are separated by an elaborate network of capillaries and both are supported by a delicate framework of reticular fibers. The epithelial cells are divided into two major groups: those that **stain** with dyes, **chromophils**; and those that **do not stain** with dyes, **chromophobes**. The chromophils are further subdivided into basophilic and acidophilic cells according to the staining properties of their secretory granules. All three cell types, basophils, acidophils and chromophobes are present in the pars distalis. **Acidophil cells** are large, round or ovoid cells (14 - 19 μm in diameter) the secretory granules of which stain with eosin (light red-pink) in standard preparations. **Basophil cells** make up a population of slightly smaller cells with basophilic staining granules. The remaining general cell type, **chromophobes**, usually are smaller and often appear confined more to the interior of the parenchymal cords. **Note**: with the development of specific antibodies to the various hormones produced by the pituitary, specific cell types within the general staining groups are readily demonstrated. Thus, if immunohistochemically stained slides are available, somatotropes and mammotrophs can be demonstrated making up acidophils. Likewise, corticotrophs, thyrotrophs and gonadotrophs make up the population of basophils.

Sketch several epithelial cords and their associated cell types. Depict the intervening capillaries between the epithelial cords.

Pars tuberalis

The pars tuberalis, if present, forms a partial sleeve of epithelial cells around the infundibular stalk. The pars tuberalis is characterized by longitudinally arranged cords of parenchymal cells separated by sinusoids. The parenchyma of the pars tuberalis is continuous with that of the pars distalis and consists of chromophobes, acidophils and basophils. Undifferentiated columnar cells also are seen.

Pars intermedia

Identify and *sketch* the position of a system of colloid-filled or empty cysts lined by a squamous to columnar epithelium that lies between the pars distalis and the pars nervosa. This region of the pituitary is the pars intermedia. The pars intermedia also contains basophils and chromophobes which encroach into the adjacent pars nervosa.

Neurohypophysis

Identify the **pars nervosa** and **infundibular stalk** segments of the neurohypophysis. The greater part of the neurohypophysis consists of **unmyelinated nerve fibers**, the cell bodies of which reside in supraoptic and paraventricular nuclei as well as other hypothalamic regions of the brain. The axons commonly contain masses of secretory material of variable size called **Herring bodies**. These can be demonstrated immunocytochemically by staining for neurophysin, a carrier protein that binds to oxytocin and vasopressin. The majority of nuclei associated with the unmyelinated axons of the pars nervosa are those of **pituicytes**. These are considered to be the equivalent to neuroglial cells of the central nervous system. Some may contain the gold-brown pigment, lipofuscin.

Table 22. Key histologic features of the classic endocrine glands.

Organ	Arrangement of cells	Cell types	Other features
Neurohypophysis	Vary in size; arranged around unmyelinated nerve fibers	Pituicytes	Herring bodies
Adenohypophysis	Irregular plates and cords	Basophils, acidophils, chromophobes	Numerous capillaries between cords
Parathyroids	Irregular plates and cords	Chief cells (majority), oxyphils (occur singly or in nests)	Abundant fat in interlobular connective tissue
Thyroid	Follicles	Follicular cells, parafollicular cells; single (adjacent to follicles) or in small interfollicular nests	Colloid in follicular lumen
Adrenal cortex:			
Zona glomerulosa	Ovoid groups or arcades	Columnar cells, occasional lipid droplets	Adjacent to capsule
Zona fasciculata	Long cords	Polyhedral cells, numerous lipid droplets	Cords of cells separated by sinusoids
Zona reticularis	Irregular, anastomosing cords	Polyhedral cells, few lipid droplets	Cords of cells separated by sinusoids
Adrenal medulla	Irregular clumps or short cords	Large, pale-staining chromaffin cells	Ganglion cells, sympathetic neurons ; sinusoids
Pineal	Poorly defined lobes, clumps, and cords	Pinealocytes, glia cells	Corpora arenacea

Eye

The eyes are made up of a series of convex surfaces with the ability to transmit and focus light on a cellular surface sensitive to the intensity and wavelength (color) of light. On exposure to light, photoreceptors in this surface produce chemical energy that is converted into the electrical energy of nerve impulses. The nerve impulses formed there are transmitted to the brain, where they are interpreted, correlated and translated into the sensation of sight. The eyes have the ability to regulate the amount of light admitted and can change their focal lengths.

Learning objectives for the eyes:

1. Know the general structure of the eye and what makes up each of its basic subcomponents.
2. Be able to recognize and describe the cell types and associated structures that form the following: corneoscleral coat, uveal layer, retina and lens.
3. List and describe the elements that form the three-neuron conducting chain of the retina and understand how the optic nerve is formed.

With the low-power objective scan the anterior portion of the eye and locate each of the following: cornea, conjunctiva, iris, anterior chamber, lens and ciliary body. Next examine each of these regions at increased magnification.

Beginning at the external surface of the **cornea,** observe that the **corneal epithelium** consists of a nonkeratinized stratified squamous epithelium five to six cells deep. The next major layer, the **substantia propria,** forms the bulk of the cornea and consists of numerous regularly arranged interlacing collagen fibers and flattened fibroblast-like cells called **keratocytes.** A thick basement membrane, homogeneous in appearance, called **Bowman's membrane,** separates the substantia propria from the corneal epithelium. Along the inner surface of the substantia propria lies another thicker homogeneous membrane, 6 - 8 μm thick, called **Descemet's membrane. Corneal endothelium** lines the inner surface of the cornea. Note its low cuboidal character.

Make a labeled sketch of a section taken through the cornea detailing its subcomponents.

Return to the low-power objective and identify a region of transition, between 1.5 mm and 2.0 mm wide, separating the cornea and sclera. This region of transition is called the **limbus.** Note that both Bowman's and Descemet's membranes end in the

limbus and that the collagen fibers and bundles of the cornea become larger in the limbus and their arrangement more irregular as they blend with those of the sclera. As Descemet's membrane ends it is replaced by an area of anastomosing trabeculae made up of collagen fibers that are covered by an attenuated endothelium. The trabeculae compartmentalize this region to form a **labyrinth of spaces** that communicate with the anterior chamber. This spongy appearing region is referred to as the **trabecular meshwork.** Between the bulk of the limbal stroma and the trabecular meshwork identify a flattened endothelium-lined canal called **Schlemm's canal.**

Return once again to low power and examine the middle vascular coat of the eye, the **uvea,** which is divided into choroid, ciliary body and iris.

The **choroid** appears as a thin, brown, highly vascular membrane that lines the interior surface of the posterior sclera. At increased magnification observe that the choroid proper consists of three regions: an **outer vessel layer,** a loose connective tissue layer filled with numerous melanocytes and numerous blood vessels; a **choriocapillary layer** made up of a network of capillaries; and the **glassy (Bruch's) membrane,** a homogeneous layer 1 - 4 μm thick, that lies between the remainder of the choroid and the pigment epithelium of the retina.

Make a detailed sketch of this region.

Move anteriorly to the **ciliary body** and observe that in section it forms a thin triangular area that consists of an inner vascular tunic and a mass of smooth muscle located immediately adjacent to the sclera. The majority of the ciliary body consists of smooth muscle, the **ciliaris muscle,** the smooth muscle cells of which are organized into regions with circular, radial and meridional orientations. Melanocytes and numerous elastic fibers form a sparse connective tissue between the muscle bundles. The internal surface is covered by **ciliary epithelium,** a continuation of the pigment epithelium of the retina that lacks photosensitive cells. The ciliary epithelium consists of an inner layer of nonpigmented cells and an outer layer of pigmented cells. This epithelium is unusual in that the cell apices of both layers are closely apposed to one another. The **outer pigmented cell layer** is continuous with the pigment epithelium in the reminder of the retina. The base of the **non-pigmented cell layer** lies immediately adjacent to the posterior chamber of the eye and its apical surface abuts the apices of cells forming the outer pigmented cell layer.

In the anterior region, the inner surface of the ciliary body is formed by 60 - 80 radially arranged, elongated ridges called **ciliary processes**. These consist of a core of highly vascularized stroma and scattered melanocytes covered by ciliary epithelium. Find and examine **zonule fibers** that extend from the basal region of the non-pigmented cell layer of the ciliary epithelium to the equator of the lens. These appear as thin homogeneous strands most of which will appear as small fragments and will not be seen in their entirety.

Make a sketch summarizing the observations of this region.

Anteriorly, the ciliary body is continuous with the **iris**, which divides the space between the lens and cornea into anterior and posterior chambers. The two chambers communicate through a space known as the **pupil**. The **stroma** of the iris consists of loose, vascular connective tissue with the collagen fibers, fibroblasts and melanocytes enveloped in an abundant transparent ground substance. Note that the **anterior surface** of the iris lacks a definite endothelial or mesothelial lining but is covered in part by a discontinuous layer of melanocytes and fibroblasts. Spaces within the stroma of the iris often appear to communicate with that of the anterior chamber. In contrast, observe that the **posterior surface** is covered by two rows of pigmented cuboidal cells that are continuous with the ciliary epithelium. Where the ciliary epithelium courses onto the posterior surface of the iris, the non-pigmented layer becomes pigmented. Cells of the outer layer in this region contain less pigment and are modified myoepithelial cells that form the **dilator** of the iris. Examine the pupillary margin of the iris for a compact bundle of smooth muscle cells that are circularly arranged around the circumference of the pupil. This is the **sphincter muscle** of the iris.

Sketch and label the histological features of the iris.

Positioned immediately behind the pupil of the iris is the **lens**. The lens is made up of a capsule, anterior lens cells and lens substance. The lens is surrounded by a homogeneous **capsule** 10 - 18 μm thick. Just anterior and posterior to the equator, examine its external surface for zonule fibers. A single layer of cuboidal cells, called **anterior lens cells**, lies immediately beneath the capsule and is restricted to the anterior surface of the lens. The posterior surface lacks an epithelium. **Lens fiber cells** constitute the bulk of lens, referred to as the **lens substance**. Lens fiber cells are elongated, light-staining cells with central elongate nuclei. Examine the equator of the lens and observe the transformation of anterior lens cells into lens fiber cells.

Sketch and label the microscopic features of the lens.

Move to the posterior region of the eye and examine the **retina**, which is the innermost layer. The posterior retina consists of an outer **pigment epithelium** and an inner **neural retina**. Under low power examine the posterior aspect of the eye and trace the retina anteriorly to a ragged margin called the **ora serrata**. Note that the retina decreases in thickness anteriorly and that the neural retina ends at the ora serrata. Return to the posterior region of the eye and examine the retina for the fovea centralis and the optic disc. The **fovea centralis** is a funnel-like depression on the posterior aspect of the retina. It measures about 1.5 mm in diameter and consists **only of cones** that are longer and thinner than elsewhere in the retina. The **optic disc** is the site of formation and exit of the optic nerve. It lacks photoreceptor cells and is the region where nerve fibers from the retina congregate before passing through the sclera to form the optic nerve.

Examine the **pigment epithelium** of the retina with the high-power objective. The pigment epithelium consists of a **simple layer** of hexagonal cells that tend to increase in diameter near the ora serrata. The cytoplasm is filled with **melanin** and **lipofuscin granules** that tend to be located apically. The basement membrane underlying the pigment epithelium contributes to the glassy (Bruch's) membrane of the choroid.

Examine the details of the neural retina and identify the following layers in order beginning at the choroid:

1. layer of rods and cones;
2. external limiting membrane;
3. outer nuclear layer;
4. outer plexiform layer;
5. inner nuclear layer;
6. inner plexiform layer;
7. ganglion cell layer;
8. layer of nerve fibers; and
9. internal limiting membrane.

When examining each of these layers understand clearly what each layer represents. The **layer of rods and cones** represents the inner and outer segments of rods and cones. The rod outer segments appear as darker-staining rods and are more numerous than the cone outer segments. The latter are larger and exhibit a conical shape. Lying between this layer and immediately adjacent the outer nuclear layer identify the **external (outer) limiting membrane**. It appears as a fine discontinuous line and is formed by junctional complexes between the scleral tips of Müller's cells and adjacent photoreceptor cells.

The **outer nuclear layer** consists of the cell bodies and nuclei of the rods and cones. The **outer plexiform layer** consists primarily of rod spherules, cone pedicles and dendrites of bipolar neurons. Nuclei and cell bodies of bipolar neurons, horizontal, amacrine and Müller's cells constitute the **inner nuclear layer**. The **inner plexiform layer** is made up of axons of bipolar neurons, dendrites of ganglion cells, and processes of amacrine cells. Ganglion cells and scattered neuroglial cells form the **ganglion cell layer**. The **nerve fiber layer** is made up primarily of unmyelinated axons from ganglion cells and processes of Müller's cells. The very thin **internal limiting membrane** is formed by the vitreal processes of Müller's cells and their basement membrane.

Make a labeled sketch of the neural retina and its relationship with the pigment epithelium.

Table 23. Key histologic features of the eye.

Region	Epithelium	Major Components	Other features
Sclera	None	Fibrous tunic	Lamina cribrosa
Cornea	Nonkeratinized stratified squamous	Bowman s membrane, substantia propria	Descemet s membrane, corneal endothelium
Choroid	None	Suprachoroid layer, choriocapillary layer, glassy membrane	Vessel layer, melanocytes
Ciliary body	Inner nonpigmented cells, outer pigmented cells	Ciliaris muscle, ciliary processes	Zonule fibers
Iris	Two layers of pigmented cells on posterior surface	Iridial stroma, sphincter muscle	Melanocytes
Neural retina	Pigment epithelium	Rods, cones, bipolar and ganglion cells	Association neurons, glia cells
Lens	Anterior lens cells	Lens fibers	Lens capsule, zonule fibers
Vitreous body	None	Hyalocytes, hyaluronic acid	Thin collagen fibers

Table 24. Contents of neural retina.

Histologic layer of retina	Principal contents
1. Layer of rods and cones	Inner and outer segments of rods and cones
2. External limiting membrane	Formed by junctional complexes between the scleral tips of M ller s cells and adjacent photoreceptor cells
3. Outer nuclear layer	Cell bodies and nuclei of rods and cones
4. Outer plexiform layer	Rod spherules, cone pedicles, dendrites of bipolar neurons, processes of horizontal cells
5. Inner nuclear layer	Nuclei of bipolar, horizontal, amacrine and M ller s cells
6. Inner plexiform layer	Axons of bipolar neurons, dendrites of ganglion cells, processes of amacrine cells
7. Ganglion cell layer	Ganglion cells, scattered neuroglial cells
8. Nerve fiber layer	Nonmyelinated nerve fibers from ganglion cells, small neuroglial cells, processes of M ller s cells
9. Internal limiting layer	Vitreal processes of M ller s cells and their basal lamina

INTERNAL EAR

The internal ear contains a sensory region and cells specialized for hearing. In this region of the ear, the mechanical vibrations of sound waves from the environment are converted to nerve impulses and relayed to the brain to be interpreted as sound. The inner ear also contains the vestibular organs that are specialized to function in balance and provide an awareness of head position and movement.

Learning objectives for the internal ear:

1. Be able to recognize and describe the histologic details of the cochlea.
2. Be able to describe and identify the cell types that make up the organ of Corti and note their relationship to the tectorial membrane.
3. Be able to recognize and describe the major subcomponents of the vestibular labyrinth: semicircular canals, utricle and saccule.
4. Be able to describe and identify the cell types that make up the cristae ampullaris, macula utriculi and macula sacculi.
5. Be able to recognize and describe the cupula cristae ampullaris and the otolithic membrane.

With the low-power objective examine a section through the cochlea, noting that it consists of a central core of spongy bone called the **modiolus** around which the cochlear canal spirals for two and three-quarter turns. Identify the **cochlear nerve** and the **spiral ganglion** within this central region of bony tissue. At increased magnification, examine a profile through the cochlear canal. Find a thin bony projection extending from the modiolus into the lumen of the cochlear canal. This is the **osseous spiral lamina**. A thin fibrous structure, the **basilar membrane**, extends from the osseous spiral lamina to the **spiral ligament**, a thickening of the periosteum on the outer bony wall of the cochlear canal. Identify an additional thin **vestibular membrane** that extends obliquely across the cochlear canal from the osseous spiral lamina to the outer wall of the cochlea. Realize that the basilar and vestibular membranes divide the cochlear canal into an upper **scala vestibuli**, an intermediate **cochlear duct** and a lower **scala tympani**. Observe that the cochlear duct is a triangular space, the floor of which is formed by the basilar membrane and its roof by the vestibular membrane. The outer wall of the cochlear duct is formed by a vascular area called the **stria vascularis**. The cochlear duct contains a region of specialized cells know as the **organ of Corti**. Note its relationship to an overlying, structureless membrane, the **tectorial membrane**. Locate and identify the following cell types and spaces that comprise the organ of Corti: **inner pillar cell**, **outer pillar cell** (these surround a small space, the inner tunnel), the **inner phalangeal cell** which supports an **inner hair cell** and **outer phalangeal cells** which support the **outer hair cells**.

Construct a labeled sketch of the cochlear duct and the organ of Corti.

Examine the section of the inner ear further for a region through one of the semicircular canals, utricle or saccule. In specific regions of each of these areas of the membranous labyrinth, the epithelium changes from simple squamous to a stratified sensory type. The sensory epithelium of each semicircular canal is restricted to the ampullary portion. The sensory epithelium together an underlying connective tissue core rich in nerve fibers forms a transverse ridge that projects into the lumen of the ampulla. Such a region is called the **cristae ampullaris**. Similar regions can be found in the utricle and saccule and are called the **macula utriculi** and **macula sacculi**, respectively. The sensory epithelium of both the cristae and maculae consist sensory hair cells and supporting (sustentacular) cells. **Hair cells** are located high within the epithelium, are light (clear) staining and have a tulip bulb shape. Adjacent dark-staining cells are the **supporting cells**. These continue laterally to the periphery of the sensory epithelium and form a simple columnar layer, the **planum semilunatum**, which lacks hair cells. Microvilli from the hair cells of the cristae ampullaris are embedded in an overlying gelatinous structure called the **cupula** that projects from the surface of the cristae into the lumen of each semicircular canal. Microvilli of hair cells from the maculae of the utricle and saccule are also embedded in an overlying gelatinous structure called the **otolithic membrane**. In addition to the gelatinous material, numerous darker-staining crystalline bodies called **otoliths (otoconia)** are suspended in this layer, hence its name.

Make a labeled sketch of one of these sensory areas.

Table 25. Key histologic features of the membranous labyrinth.

Subdivision	Receptor region	Neuroepithelium	Other features
Semicircular canals (3)	Cristae ampullaris	Type I and II hair cells	Cupula
Utricle (1)	Macula (of utricle)	Type I and II hair cells	Otolithic membrane
Saccule (1)	Macula (of saccule)	Type I and II hair cells	Otolithic membrane
Cochlear duct (1)	Organ of Corti	Inner hair cells, outer hair cells	Tectorial membrane, basilar membrane, inner and outer phalangeal cells

Appendix Table 1. Key histologic features that distinguish between cartilages, bone and tendon.

Tissue	Arrangement of cells and lacunae	Other features
Hyaline cartilage	Glasslike matrix; lacunae randomly distributed, slitlike in appearance near perichondrium	Isogenous groups; territorial matrix
Elastic cartilage	Matrix more fibrous in appearance; elastic fibers (need to be stained selectively)	Large isogenous groups
Decalcified bone	Lacunae show organization within lamellae of osteons; haversian canals and their contents	Tide marks; bone marrow; canaliculi
Ground bone	Haversian systems obvious; interstitial and circumferential lamellae	Canaliculi and lacunae obvious
Fibrocartilage	Dense fibrous connective tissue a dominant feature with a small amount of ground substance; lacunae few in number and often aligned in rows between collagenous fibers	Round chondrocytes
Tendon	Fibroblast nuclei are densely stained and elongate; lie in parallel rows between collagen fibers	Lacunae absent

Appendix Table 2. Key histologic features that distinguish between connective tissue, muscle and nerve.

Tissue	Characteristics of nuclei	Shape and orientation of cells and fibers	Additional features
Loose areolar connective tissue	Fibroblast nuclei stain either intensely or lightly, appear scattered within the extracellular matrix	Fibroblasts and extracellular fibers are randomly orientated; extracellular fibers stain intensely	Scattered fat cells, adipose tissue
Peripheral nerve	Numerous Schwann cell nuclei, stain lightly, may be stippled in appearance, oriented in same direction	Schwann cells (nuclei) lie parallel to axis cylinders	Undulating or wavy appearance of discrete nerve bundles; limited by perineurium; nodes of Ranvier and axis cylinders may be visible
Smooth muscle	Single, oval-shaped, light-staining	Small, spindle-shaped cells; single central nucleus; well-stained cytoplasm, nuclei oriented in same direction	Cells organized into sheets or layers; scant intervening connective tissue
Dense regular connective tissue	Dense-staining; elongate fibroblast nuclei organized in rows	Large, dense-staining collagen fibers arranged in parallel; fibers and fibroblasts orderly arranged in same direction	Dense, uniform or organized general appearance
Skeletal muscle	Numerous light-staining peripheral nuclei within each cell	Cells arranged in same direction per fascicle; striations of cell visible in longitudinal section	Connective tissue visible around individual cells, organizes several cells into fascicles
Cardiac muscle	Usually a single, large light-staining central nucleus; occasional cell shows two nuclei	Branching cells oriented in the same direction as others in a specific layer; faint cross striations as for skeletal muscle	Intercalated discs
Dense irregular connective tissue	Dense-staining, fibroblast nuclei without organization	Large, dense-staining interwoven collagen fibers without organization, fibroblasts scattered without orientation	Dense, unorganized general appearance

Appendix Table 3. Key histologic features that distinguish major glandular structures.

Organ	Secretory units	Ductal system	Other features
Parotid gland	All acini (alveoli) and tubules are serous	Prominent intercalated ducts; intralobular duct system prominent	Numerous fat cells scattered throughout parotid
Pancreas	Acini and tubules are comprised of pyramidal shaped cells; zymogen granules prominent	Centroacinar cells, prominent intralobular ducts	Islets of Langerhans
Lacrimal gland	All acini and tubules are serous; cells low columnar	Inconspicuous	Occasional fat cells; gland small in size
Submandibular gland	Most acini and tubules are serous; a few mucous tubules capped with serous demilunes	Very prominent intralobular duct system, especially striated ducts; numerous profiles in each lobule	Occasional fat cells
Sublingual gland	Mucous and serous acini and tubules equal in abundance; mucous tubules capped by serous demilunes	Intralobular duct system not prominent	Occasional fat cells
Thyroid	Large follicles filled with homogeneous colloid	Absent	Nests of parafollicular (C) cells between follicles
Mammary gland, lactating	Large, expanded alveoli that contain a thin secretion	Ducts visible in interlobular connective tissue	Lobulated
Mammary gland, non lactating	Alveoli poorly developed	Intralobular and interlobular ducts visible	Lobulated, loose connective tissue and fat abundant
Parathyroid gland	Irregular chords of chief cells; individual or clumps of oxyphil cells	Absent	Abundant fat cells in gland and surrounding connective tissue
Adenohypophysis	Irregular cords or clumps of epithelial cells; basophils, acidophils, chromophobes	Absent	Abundant capillaries separating epithelial cords
Adrenal	Cortex: cells arranged into epithelial cords separated by sinusoids; three zones (glomerulosa, fasciculata, reticularis) Medulla: large, light staining chromaffin cells	Absent	Cortex: dark-staining Medulla: light-staining; obvious dilated veins in medulla

Appendix Table 4. Key histologic features that distinguish solid, gland-like structures.

Organ	Secretory units/tubules	Ductal system	Other features
Ovary	Ovarian follicles in cortex	Absent	Surface covering mesothelium; cortex; medulla of connective tissue and blood vessels
Kidney	Parenchyma consists of tubules forming nephrons; large, scattered, renal corpuscles	Large, light-staining collecting ducts in medulla and medullary rays	Cortex: dark-staining tubules Medulla: light-staining tubules arranged in parallel
Testis	Seminiferous tubules, spermatogenic cells	Rete testis, efferent ductules	Tunica albuginea, septa, interstitial cells
Liver	Hepatic lobules	Interlobular bile ducts	Portal areas containing branches of bile duct, hepatic artery, portal vein, and lymphatic vessel

Appendix Table 5. Key histologic features that distinguish large tubular structures.

Organ	Epithelial lining	Muscle coats	Special features
Esophagus	Nonkeratinized stratified squamous	Prominent muscularis mucosae; muscularis externa of inner circular and outer longitudinal layers; skeletal (upper), mixed smooth and skeletal (middle), smooth (lower)	Glands present in submucosa; may occur in lamina propria at distal and proximal ends
Small intestine	Simple columnar, striated border; scattered , goblet cells	Muscularis mucosae and externa, inner circular, outer longitudinal layers of smooth muscle	Villi; intestinal glands; Brunner s glands in submucosa of duodenum; Peyer s patches in ileum
Colon	Simple columnar, striated border; abundant goblet cells	Same as above but outer longitudinal layer of muscularis externa is thinner except for taeniae coli	Villi absent, smooth luminal surface, intestinal glands
Trachea, bronchi	Ciliated pseudostratified columnar; goblet cells	Thin muscularis mucosae	Rings of hyaline cartilage
Aorta and major conducting arteries	Endothelium	Tunica media dominant layer; smooth muscle and elastic laminae	Lumen usually circular in outline; vasa vasorum
Vena cava and large veins	Endothelium	Tunica adventitia is main layer; collagen and elastic fibers, smooth muscle cells	Lumen is often irregular in shape
Vagina	Nonkeratinized stratified squamous	Lacks muscularis mucosae; coat of inner circular and outer longitudinal smooth muscle	Prominent venous plexus in lamina propria; vagina lacks glands

Appendix Table 6. Key histologic features that distinguish small tubular structures.

Organs	Epithelial lining	Smooth muscle coats	Special features
Distributing arteries	Endothelium	Tunica media prominent	Internal and external elastic laminae
Oviduct	Ciliated simple columnar, peg cells	Inner circular, outer longitudinal layers	Plicae
Ureter	Transitional	Proximal 2/3 , inner longitudinal, outer circular layers; Distal 1/3 , inner longitudinal, middle circular, outer longitudinal layers	Stellate lumen
Appendix	Simple columnar with striated border, goblet cells	Inner circular, outer longitudinal layers, muscularis mucosae present	Lacks villi; much nodular and diffuse lymphatic tissue; small diameter relative to intestines
Vas deferens	Pseudostratified columnar	Inner longitudinal, middle circular, outer longitudinal layers	Small irregular lumen bounded by a thick coat of smooth muscle

Appendix Table 7. Key histologic features that distinguish major abrupt junctions.

Junction	Changes in epithelium	Other features
Olfactory: respiratory junction of nasal cavity	Olfactory **to** ciliated pseudostratified columnar with goblet cells	Thick lamina propria containing nerves, serous glands, and venous sinuses to a thin, vascular lamina propria
Oropharynx: nasopharynx junction at edge of soft palate	Nonkeratinized stratified squamous **to** ciliated pseudostratified columnar with goblet cells	Central core of skeletal muscle, mucous/seromucous glands in connective tissue underlying epithelium
Integument: oral mucosal junction at vermilion border of lip	Typical thin skin with hair follicles, sebaceous glands and sweat glands **to** a thick, nonkeratinized stratified squamous	Typical dermis of thin skin to a thick submucosa with tall connective tissue papillae extending into the oral epithelium; labial salivary glands; skeletal muscle core between skin and oral mucosa
Rectoanal junction	Simple columnar with striated border and goblet cells **to** nonkeratinized stratified squamous epithelium	Intestinal glands and muscularis mucosae of rectum **are lost** at rectoanal junction
Esophageal-gastric junction	Thick, nonkeratinized stratified squamous **to** tall simple columnar	Branched tubular glands of esophagus **to** gastric pits and simple branched tubular cardiac glands of the stomach
Gastrointestinal junction	Tall simple columnar **to** simple columnar with striated (microvillus) border and goblet cells	Gastric pits, pyloric glands **to** villi, intestinal glands, Brunner s glands in submucosa
Vaginal-cervical junction	Nonkeratinized stratified squamous **to** tall, light-staining simple columnar	Coarse, vascular lamina propria devoid of glands, muscularis of smooth muscle **to** dense connective tissue wall containing cervical glands, Nabothian cysts

Low columnar, 9
Lungs,
    alveoli of, 64, 65
    bronchi of, 62-65
    bronchioles of, 64, 65
Lunule, 48
Lymph capillaries, 40
Lymph nodes, 42, 43, 46
    sinuses of, 43, 46
    structure of, 42, 43, 46
    vascularization of, 43
Lymph vascular system, 40
Lymphatic nodules, 42, 44
Lymphatic organs, 42-46
    lymph nodes, 42, 43, 46
    spleen, 43-46
    thymus, 45, 46
    tonsils, 42, 46
Lymphatic sinuses, 43, 46
Lymphatic trunks, 40
Lymphocytes,
    characteristics of, 31
    classification of, 31
    large, 31, 32, 45
    medium, 45
    small, 31, 32, 45

Macroglia, 27
Macrophages,
    alveolar, 65
    connective tissue, 17, 18
    hepatic, 60
Macula densa, 67
Macula sacculi, 89, 90
Macula utriculi, 89, 90
Major salivary glands, 51, 52
Male reproductive system, 70-74
Mammary glands, 80
Mammotrophs, 83
Marginal sinus, 43
Marginal zone, 44
Marrow,
    structure of, 32
    types of, 32
Mast cells, 17, 18
Matrix, 19
    of bone, 20
    of cartilage, 19
Mature follicle, 75, 77
Mediastinum testis, 70
Medium veins, 39, 41
Medulla,
    adrenal, 82, 84
    of hair, 48
    of lymph node, 43, 46
    renal, 67, 68

of thymus, 45, 46
Medullary collecting ducts, 67, 68
Medullary sinus of lymph node, 43
Megakaryocyte, 34, 36
Meissner's corpuscles, 27, 48
Meissner's plexus, 52, 54, 55
Melanin granules, 47
Melanocytes, 47
Membranous urethra, 68, 69
Merkel's cells, 47
Mesothelium, 8
Metamyelocyte, 33, 36
Microcytic erythrocytes, 30
Microglia, 27
Microtome, 4
Microvilli, 10, 11
Mixed gland, 14
Modiolus, 89
Molecular layer, 28
Monocytes, 31, 32
Mononuclear leukocytes, 31
Motor end-plate, 27
Mounted sections, 4
Mucosa, 50, 52
    of digestive tract, 50-56
    of large intestine, 55
    of small intestine, 54
    of stomach, 53, 57
Mucous cells, 13
Mucous membrane, 50
Mucous neck cells, 53, 57
M ller's cells, 87, 88
Multicellular exocrine glands, 12
Multipolar neurons, 25
Muscle,
    cardiac, 23, 24
    skeletal, 23, 24
    smooth, 23, 24
Myofibrils, 23
Muscular arteries, 38, 41
Muscularis externa, 52, 57, 58
    of esophagus, 53, 57
    of large intestine, 55, 58
    of small intestine, 55, 58
    of stomach, 54, 57
Muscularis mucosae, 52
    of small intestine, 54, 58
    of stomach, 54, 57
Myelin sheath, 26
Myelinated fiber, 26
Myeloblasts, 33, 36
Myelocytes, 33, 36
Myenteric plexus, 54, 55, 58
Myocardium, 37
Myoepithelial cells,
    of salivary glands, 51

of sweat glands, 49

Nail,
    bed, 48
    matrix, 48
    plate, 48
    root, 48
Nasal cavity, 61
Nasopharynx, 61
Negative Golgi, 17
Nephron, 66
Nerves,
    cells of, 25
    fibers of, 26
Neural retina, 86, 88
Neurilemma, 26
Neurofibrils, 25
Neuroglia, 27
Neurohypophysis, 82-84
Neurokeratin, 26
Neurons, 7, 25-29
Neurophysin, 83
Neutrophils,
    characteristics of, 30, 32
    formation of, 33, 34, 36
Nipple, 80
Nissl substance, 25
Nodes of Ranvier, 26
Nodular lymphatic tissue, 42-46
Nonkeratinized stratified squamous
epithelium, 9, 11
Nonpyramidal cells of cerebral
cortex, 28
Normoblasts, 33
Nucleolus, 6
Nucleus, 6

Odontoblasts, 52
Olfactory epithelium, 61
Olfactory cilia, 61
Olfactory knob, 61
Olfactory neurons, 61
Oligodendrocytes, 27, 29
Oocyte, 6, 75-77
Optic disc, 86
Optic nerve, 86
Ora serrata, 86
Oral cavity, 50
Oral mucosa, 50
Organ of Corti, 89
Organelles, 7
Osseous spiral lamina, 89
Ossification, 20-22
    endochondral, 21, 22
    intramembranous, 21
Osteoblasts, 20, 21

Printed in the United Kingdom
by Lightning Source UK Ltd.
119584UK00001B/46